HANDBOOK OF
STUTTERING
THERAPY
FOR THE
SCHOOL CLINICIAN

HANDBOOK OF STUTTERING THERAPY FOR THE SCHOOL CLINICIAN

William R. Leith, PhD
Wayne State University

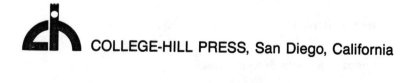
COLLEGE-HILL PRESS, San Diego, California

College-Hill Press, Inc.
4284 41st Street
San Diego, California 92105

Library of Congress Cataloging in Publication Data
Leith, William, 1927–

    Handbook of stuttering therapy for the school clinician.

      Bibliography: p.
      Includes index.
      1. Stuttering in children—Treatment—Handbooks, manuals, etc. 2. Speech therapy—
Handbooks, manuals, etc. 3. Stuttering—Treatment—Handbooks, manuals, etc. I. Title.
RJ496.S8L45   1984   618.92'855406   84-12698

ISBN 0-933014-29-5

Printed in the United States of America.

To all clinicians who are providing therapy
for persons who stutter
and to
all persons who stutter
who are receiving therapy

CONTENTS

Dedication

Preface

Acknowledgments

SECTION II: STUTTERING THERAPY

Appendices

Indices

PREFACE

Of all the disorders of communication, none has been as thoroughly researched as the phenomenon of stuttering and none continues to be as baffling. We continue to attempt to resolve the stuttering riddle but, regardless of the claims of some, the riddle has not been solved. We are still searching for a cure and, in the meantime, we are still searching for effective and efficient treatment procedures.

The speech clinician who provides the vast majority of the clinical services to persons who stutter is the school speech clinician. And yet the treatment programs that are available, written in enough detail that they can be applied by a clinician, have not addressed the logistical problems faced by the school clinician. Treatment programs commonly require two or three lengthy individual therapy sessions each week. Others rely on expensive clinical equipment. Both of these factors militate against their application in a school environment where time is precious and budgets are limited. In many instances school clinicians are left to fend for themselves when confronted with a client who stutters.

Having worked closely with clinical programs in a number of school districts in Indiana, Ohio, and Michigan, and presenting workshops for other districts throughout the country, it became increasingly apparent to me that the school clinician, who needs the most resources to turn to, has, in fact, the fewest. Her clinical problems and needs have been all but ignored. She is expected to adapt time-consuming and equipment-dependent treatment programs to the limitations imposed by the school clinical environment. This situation provided the impetus for my writing this book: to provide the school speech clinician with a treatment program specifically designed for the school working environment. Recognizing that there are many factors influencing the provision of services in the schools, I worked closely with school speech clinicians in the Detroit and Cleveland public schools. Their input was crucial in making the therapy and the book practical for the school clinical environment. The treatment program has been presented through workshops and short courses for several years and feedback from clinicians who have used the program over the years has also influenced the development of the book.

This book was written by a clinician to a clinician. It is a sharing of clinical expertise which was developed during 30 years of working with stutterers. The treatment program is designed specifically for the school clinician and I hope you find it applicable to your unique clinical needs.

William R. Leith

Acknowledgments

I am indebted to numerous people for their assistance in the development of this book. I particularly thank all the school speech/language clinicians who reviewed the manuscript and offered suggestions to make the book more applicable to the unique clinical environment found in the schools. Those clinicians in the Detroit public schools I thank are Ted Mandell, Beverly Barlow, Linda Jacobs, Ann James, and April Marcus. In the Cleveland public schools I extend my thanks to Susan Braun, Vicki Brown, and Jana Sward.

Very special help was provided by Karen Schmanski, speech/language clinician at Bon Secours Hospital, Grosse Pointe, Michigan; Denise Dinan-Panico, speech/language clinician in the South Lake schools, St. Clair Shores, Michigan; Dr. Mae Taylor, specialist in communication disorders, Utah State Board of Education; Paul DeVreugd, clinical supervisor, Medi-Speech, Inc, Troy Michigan; and Dr. Mary Jane Dettman, private practice in Cleveland, Ohio. I especially appreciate the help of all the students in my undergraduate and graduate courses in stuttering at Wayne State University who were subjected to the manuscript for a period of 2 years.

Finally, I thank CVR for teaching me the importance of the clinican and therapy in my chosen profession.

Section I:
Basic Principles
of Treatment

Chapter 1

Introduction: Stuttering Therapy in the Schools

FACTORS INFLUENCING STUTTERING THERAPY IN THE SCHOOLS

This book is directed not only to the speech/language pathologist providing services in a school environment, but also to the student in training who plans to work in the schools. Before we proceed, let us establish some terminology for our discussions. In this book I will refer to the speech/language pathologist as the "speech clinician" or "clinician." I will also refer to the clinician as "she" since a majority of clinicians are female. I have not overlooked the male clinicians. They are an extremely important part of this special group, the school clinicians, and can often work with a male stutterer more effectively than can a female clinician. In terms of the client, I will refer to the stuttering client as "he" since a majority of stutterers are male. These terms should help prevent confusion as to whether we are discussing the client or the clinician.

The school clinician is faced with a uniquely demanding environment in which to provide therapy for the client who stutters. The clinician's schedule is such that most treatment programs for stuttering can not be applied as intended, thus negating their effectiveness. Although there is no typical school environment, most present the following factors the clinician must deal with in terms of providing clinical services: time constraints, large case loads, limited contact with parents, providing services in a unique peer environment, and, in many instances, lack of client motivation.

The school clinician typically provides clinical services to a large number of clients who have a wide variety of communication problems. Due to the large number of clients, the amount of clinical time available for each client is limited. In addition to the large case loads, the time available for therapy is further reduced by the record keeping and other forms of paper work required by the school district. This "paper work" time, plus the large number of clients assigned to the clinician, present some very real problems in terms of scheduling time for delivery of services to the clients.

With the above constraints, the school clinician must provide most of her services in a group setting. She may be able to arrange her schedule in order to provide some individual therapy but this is the exception rather than the rule. This is not to say that group therapy is not an effective treatment procedure, but the stuttering treatment programs currently available to the clinician are based on several individual therapy sessions with the client each week.

Considering the above-mentioned time limitations, the clinician also has limited time for parent conferences. Further, in that the parents are usually not directly involved in the treatment program since they do not have to bring their child to therapy, additional problems are created in terms of making contacts with parents, getting them involved in the treatment program, and developing this parental clinical support system. Of course, parental involvement also depends on their attitudes. If the parents are cooperative, the clinician can, according to her own time constraints, involve the parents in the therapy. However, if the parents are not cooperative, the clinician must work with the child independently in the school environment. It is important to note that, in most instances, the parents have not initiated the treatment program by requesting therapy. If the parents have requested therapy, there is some indication of interest and possible involvement on their part. There are also those parents who are truly interested in their child's therapy but who are unavailable because of their work schedules or other factors. There are four possible parental situations that the clinician may face: cooperative and available parents, cooperative but unavailable parents, uncooperative but available parents, and uncooperative and unavailable parents. These situations are dealt with according to the clinician's time constraints and the parents' attitudes.

The school clinician also works in a unique social environment. Her clients are functioning in a peer society within the school during the time they are receiving therapy. Unlike the services offered by an agency where the child is removed from the peer environment and taken to the agency, the school clinician provides her services within the peer environment. The peer society exerts great influence on its members. This influence takes many forms and the forms change according to the age group in the peer society. The peer pressures in elementary schools are different from those in junior high schools, which are again different from the pressures in high schools. Having a student leave a classroom of peers to go for speech therapy may indeed have some negative influence on the student's attitude toward therapy.

There is also the important factor of the child's motivation for therapy. If a child asks his parents if he can get help for his stuttering or if he approaches the speech clinician, we can assume that the child has some motivation to deal with the stuttering. However, this is the exception rather than the rule in the schools. In most instances, the child is referred for therapy; someone other than the child has decided that he should have therapy and he then becomes involved in therapy with no motivation to work on his stuttering. He may indeed be cooperative, attending therapy and doing what is asked in therapy, but have no motivation to work on the stuttering outside the therapy environment. There is a significant difference between cooperation and motivation, and motivation in one form or another is essential for successful therapy.

THE COGNITIVE BEHAVIOR TREATMENT PROGRAM FOR STUTTERING

For a treatment program to be applied effectively in the school environment, it must address the factors set forth above. The treatment program presented in this book is specifically designed to deal with these issues so that it is compatible with the clinical environment in the schools.

Time Constraints

The treatment program is based on an average of two short therapy sessions per week and a minimum of individual therapy contact. The only time individual therapy may be called for is in the first stage of therapy, getting the new speech behavior to occur. Once this has been accomplished, usually within six therapy sessions, the client should be seen in group therapy. The minimal demands for individual therapy and clinical contact time will relieve the clinician of many scheduling problems. She will not have to juggle her schedule in order to provide the stutterer with several therapy sessions each week or with long-term individual therapy. This increased flexibility in her clinical time should also be of benefit to her other clients since she should have more time for therapy planning, for therapy contact, or for parent conferences if this is part of her treatment program.

Group Therapy

The treatment program presented here is based essentially on a group therapy approach. It can be administered in individual therapy but is usually more effective when applied in the group therapy environment. The flexibility of the treatment program provides the clinician with a choice of therapy modes: individual sessions, group sessions, or any combination of the two. Her decision will be influenced by her comfort in working in a group setting, the sizes of her groups, the personality of the client, the client's cognitive set, or other factors. However, group therapy has many advantages in stuttering treatment that individual therapy cannot offer and, in certain stages of treatment, group therapy should be the therapy mode of choice, not a forced alternative. Because of the importance of group therapy in this treatment program, an entire chapter is devoted to operational aspects of group therapy.

Lack of Parental Involvement

Since the school clinician has limited parental contact and involvement, the treatment program provides the clinician with methods for enlisting parental participation, either direct or indirect, in the treatment program. In the event that parental involvement is not possible, the clinician is given means to compensate for this by developing other clinical support systems. This includes working with teachers and other people in the client's life as well as with the other members of the client's therapy group. Special emphasis is given to means of generalizing the new speech behavior in the absence of parental support.

Peer Pressure

Since the stuttering treatment is provided within the peer environment in the school, the treatment program takes this factor into account. The clinician is given strategies to deal with negative peer pressure and to utilize positive peer pressure as part of the treatment procedure. Clinical procedures include working on the stutterer's cognitive set with special emphasis on understanding listener's reactions to his stuttering and on improving his self-concept and self-confidence. Other strategies include utilizing the positive peer responses in group therapy to off-set negative peer responses he may encounter in the classroom and formation of a support system within the school environment.

Client Motivation

In that the success of any stuttering treatment program is dependent on the motivation the client has to work on his stuttering, the program provides specific ways to deal with the problem. The clinician is provided with specific methods to create and maintain motivation in clients. This is especially important when the clinician is working with the very young stutterer or with any stutterer who is in therapy, not because he requested it, but because his parents or a teacher felt he should be receiving therapy.

HANDBOOK ORIENTATION AND ORGANIZATION

The cognitive behavior stuttering treatment program makes use of the clinical skills of the clinician and allows her to make clinical judgments based on her professional training and experience. It does not view the clinician as a "technician," applying a series of regimented steps or procedures where she is allowed no clinical judgments in the treatment program, but as a professional clinician who is capable of making decisions and judgments and able to carry on a comprehensive treatment program.

The therapy program is developed in three parts in the first section of the book. The parts are the clinician/client interactions in therapy, behavioral and cognitive aspects of stuttering which underlie the treatment program, and a cognitive behavior form of group therapy. The clinical interactions are developed in chapters 2 and 3. Cognitive learning and operant procedures are discussed and a basic therapeutic clinical interaction concept, the clinical interaction model, is developed from these learning orientations. The clinical interaction model represents all clinical interactions between the clinician and the client, parents, significant other, teachers, or any other persons involved in the treatment program. It forms the foundation of therapy.

The phenomenon of stuttering is discussed in chapters 4, 5, and 6. The discussion includes not only the behaviors that are directly or indirectly associated with stuttering, but also the effects that stuttering has on the cognitive sets of the stutterer and his parents and how these sets effect therapy. The discussion is not meant to be a definitive treatise on stuttering but rather a view of the phenomenon which supports the cognitive behavior treatment program. This part concludes by considering some behavioral or cognitive factors which might interfere with the treatment program.

The final part, chapter 7, presents a form of group therapy which is based on the cognitive behavior approach to therapy. Both the criteria for group organization and guidelines for the operation of this form of group therapy are included in the chapter.

The reader who has an extensive background in the area of stuttering may choose to read only selected chapters in this section. However, it is recommended that chapter 2 be included in the readings since the clinical interaction model forms the base of clinical interactions in the treatment procedure.

The treatment program is presented in the final section of the book. Chapter 8 provides the reader with an overview of the total treatment program so the relationships between the various steps in treatment can be seen more clearly. Diagrams are also provided illustrating the interactions between the clinician and the client in all phases of the treatment program.

Detailed presentations of the treatment process for stutterers from 2 to 8 years of age and stutterers from 9 years of age through adulthood are to be found in chapters 9 and 10. Although the two treatment programs differ slightly in terms of concepts, they both follow the principles of cognitive behavior stuttering therapy presented in chapter 8.

Each of the treatment programs is complete within itself and enough detail is provided to minimize the need for the clinician to go to different sections of the book in order to apply the program. However, if a clinician feels that she would like additional information on a clinical concept, page references are provided which direct her to the part of the book where the concept was discussed in detail.

Each treatment program is viewed as being made up of both pretherapy and therapy procedures. Pretherapy procedures include the initial evaluation, the conference with the parents, and, with the older stutterers, pretherapy informational meetings with the client. Therapy procedures include getting the new behavior to occur, stabilizing the new behavior, generalizing the new behavior, and maintaining the new behavior. As each therapy procedure is presented, the reader is first given an overview of the clinical activities in this step of therapy followed by a detailed presentation of the activities.

With this organization, the clinician is provided with three levels of detail of the therapy procedure: detailed clinical activities within each step of therapy, an overview of clinical activities within each step, and an overview of the total treatment procedure. The material was organized this way in order to adapt it to clinicians with varying degrees of clinical experience with stuttering. It not only provides the detailed procedures for less experienced clinicians and students in training, but also broader and more general guidelines for more experienced clinicians. The guidelines for the experienced clinician will increase the efficiency of her therapy time by eliminating the necessity of going through clinical details she is already familiar with.

If, as you read, you get the feeling that I have a tendency to repeat concepts, you are correct. I have found over the years, in both my therapy and my teaching, that an ounce of redundancy is worth a pound of reminding. Even though a concept may be repeated several times in the book, each presentation is from a slightly different stand point. You will also note that concepts are discussed in detail in the first section of the book and are then repeated in an abbreviated form when they are part of a therapy procedure. The highlights are presented to remind you of important points to remember. Again, reference page numbers are provided if you need to review the discussion of the concept to refresh your memory.

Chapter 2

Principles of Cognitive Behavior Therapy

THE COGNITIVE BEHAVIORAL ORIENTATION

Because of the nature of this book, the presentation of cognitive behavior therapy which follows is an abbreviated form. A detailed presentation of this approach to therapy is contained in the book *Handbook of Clinical Methods in Communication Disorders* (Leith, 1984). Cognitive behavior therapy is the core of the stuttering treatment program presented here and it is strongly recommended that you review the material contained in the above reference for a more comprehensive understanding of the concept.

As we discuss the development and treatment of stuttering we approach it both from a cognitive and a behavioral point of view. Our cognitive behavior approach utilizes concepts from cognitive learning theory as well as from operant conditioning. It is important to recognize the interaction between cognitive learning and "noncognitive" conditioning and that the client's cognitions, his thinking processes, are an integral part of both the development and the treatment of stuttering. The cognitive and behavioral influence in the development of stuttering are presented in chapters to follow. In this chapter the concepts involved in cognitive behavior therapy are developed.

Cognitive behavior modification, as a specialized area of behavior therapy, was introduced in the later 1970's (Meichenbaum, 1977). In our discussion of the role of cognition in therapy, we consider cognitive involvement both of the client and of the clinician. The client must perceive and comprehend all of the information presented to him by the clinician. The clinician must also be involved in therapy on a cognitive level, evaluating the client's responses, determining an appropriate response to the client's behavior, changing the clinical strategy if the client fails to respond or comprehend, and so forth. And, particularly with the stutterer, the clinician must be aware of the client's cognitive set, that is, his attitudes, emotions, and needs. The cognitive set is an important part of our therapy and we will be dealing with it in each phase of therapy.

We start our discussion of our cognitive behavior therapy by considering some basic learning theories and concepts. However, before we discuss them, it is important to clarify the following terminology. In operant conditioning, the terms "reinforce" and "punish" may be confusing to some and create misunderstanding in others. This is particularly true of the term "punish." The terms "reward" and "penalty," often used as synonyms for "reinforce" and "punish," are the terms we will use as we discuss operant procedures since the terms are clearer in meaning to people not familiar with operant conditioning. This is an important consideration for the school clinician who must communicate with other professionals, such as administrators, teachers, occupational therapists, physical therapists, and counselors, who may not have a clear understanding of the terms "reinforce" and "punish." There is also the negative connotation of the term "punish." I have found that the term "penalize" does not seem to have the same degree of negative impact.

When we apply a reward or a penalty, we create different attitudes in our clients, different clinical cognitive sets. With a reward, the client's attitude is positive and he performs those behaviors which yield more rewards. When penalty is used, the client's attitude is negative in that he avoids performing the behavior that results in penalty. He will perform some other behavior so he will not be penalized. These different cognitive sets are very important since we will be using both in our therapy. To identify them we will use the terms "approach motivation" and "avoidance motivation."

When a client's behavior is followed by something positive (reward), the client acquires approach motivation. He is motivated to perform the behavior more often in order to achieve more of the reward. If the client's behavior is followed by something negative (penalty), the client acquires avoidance motivation. He is motivated to avoid the penalty by not performing the behavior as often. We are now ready to discuss two of the more important learning concepts.

LEARNING ORIENTATIONS

Our treatment program will utilize concepts and principles primarily from two learning approaches, cognitive and behavioral. We will discuss each rather briefly. For a broader and deeper understanding of the approaches you are referred to the References and Recommended Reading section.

Cognitive

Cognition is a complex phenomenon. It is involved in the reception of information, the thinking about the information, and planning the response to the information. Those aspects of cognition most important to the speech clinician are memory and problem solving.

The two types of memory are long-term and short-term. Long-term memory implies that information is retained over long periods of time. For it to be retained, it is rehearsed often, for example, giving your name and telephone number or using information received in a class during training. You may have remembered it long enough to pass tests but do you still remember it? It depends on how often you use it and recall it. If the information is not recalled periodically, it is "forgotten." Short-term memory is for information to be retained briefly and then discarded. It is our short-term memory that allows us to remember a telephone number long enough to dial it, or to remember the names of people at social functions, or where we put our coffee cup (a problem with many of us).

We use both forms of memory in our therapy. When we teach a new behavior or concept, we depend on the client to remember this for an extended period of time. The lack of long-term memory creates problems in our therapy. If the client does not remember things from one therapy session to the next, each clinical session has to start from the beginning of therapy, each session being a new experience for the client.

Short-term memory also has an impact on our therapy. We often give our clients instructions for performing a task or a behavior. If this information is not retained long enough to influence the performance of the task or behavior, we have a serious problem in providing therapy.

Memory is also the source of the stutterer's cognitive set; his attitudes, beliefs, emotions, concepts, and so forth. The stutterer remembers his failures, his unsuccessful attempts to change his speech, his embarrassment, the penalties he has received. He develops a negative cognitive set based on these memories and this set becomes a very important factor that we must deal with in our therapy.

Another aspect of cognition that influences our therapy is problem solving through insight. This is the sudden recognition of a solution to a problem. It is the sudden realization of the relationships between factors or bits of information. There is a word game that is based on problem solving through insight. Examine the following word game and see if you can figure out a special meaning hidden in each. The answers will be given later in the chapter.

1. SPEDEFECTECH
2. EYE CON
               TACT

3. | STUTTERING |

We present our client with "problems" to which they must find solutions. For example, we model a behavior and they must find a way to imitate it. We give them information on how to slow down the rate of speech and they have to figure out how to do it. They must integrate all of this information, see the interrelationships, and gain insight into the "problem" before they can produce the behavior correctly. Consider the client who is given the rules concerning phonology. He must "understand" the rules before he can apply them to his speech. In other words, he must see the relationships between the rules and his speech (gain "insight") before there is a change in the speech behaviors. We might view this as verbal comprehension. Our client can only comprehend what we tell him after he has compared it with his long-term memories of past experiences and understands the relationships between what we said and what he has experienced. He must understand not only the words he hears, but also the relationships between them and the concepts they convey.

Behavioral

We will now consider operant or instrumental conditioning. The important thing to remember here is that the learning that occurs is dependent on the consequence of the behavior, what happens after the behavior occurs. If the person views the consequence as positive, the behavior has been rewarded and there is an increased probability that it will occur again. However, if the person views the consequence as negative, there is a decreased probability of future occurrence of the behavior since it was penalized.

As can be seen, we learn both through rewards and through penalties. If there is reward each time we perform a behavior, we quickly earn to perform the behavior more often in order to get the reward. However, if the result of our performing a behavior is penalty, we stop performing the behavior so that we can avoid the penalty.

Operant conditioning procedures are used in almost all therapy provided by speech clinicians. Some programs are reward oriented while others are penalty oriented. But, in the main, most clinical applications of these principles are combined so that the client receives both reward and penalty. Correct speech behaviors are encouraged through rewards while incorrect speech behaviors are discouraged through penalty.

When we use penalty we provide the client with negative "feedback" that indicates that the behavior he performed is not correct, not acceptable, or not performed as well as we know he can do. We must respond to the client both positively and negatively in order to provide him with some guidance as he goes through the various steps of therapy.

Now, we need to extend this a bit further and understand that there are two forms of rewards and two forms of penalty. The most common form of reward is to present the client with something he likes. If he likes chocolate, he is rewarded when he receives chocolate candy after performing a behavior. If he has learned the value of a token in a token economy, the token is also rewarding. This is a positive reward. Now let us turn the concept around. Let us now consider the removal of something that he feels is a penalty. Consider, for example, the child who is at the early stages of stuttering and blinks his eyes during a stuttering block. The eye blink interrupts the stuttering block and terminates it. The eye blink caused the penalty of stuttering to be removed. The eye blink is then negatively rewarded in that it was instrumental in removing the penalizing behavior of stuttering. This is how secondary mannerisms are learned.

We had also mentioned that there are two forms of penalty. We can view them in the same way, the presenting of something negative or the removal of something positive. We penalize by application when we tell the client he did a poor job, or make him repeat words he did not produce correctly. Penalty by removal would consist of taking away a toy he was playing with instead of attending to therapy, or removing a token if we are using a token economy.

In that we are dealing with stutterers, we should view penalty from the standpoint of avoidance conditioning. This means that the stutterer has received so much penalty from his stuttering that he will do anything to avoid it. His entire life revolves around avoiding stuttering. This cognitive set has a profound effect on our therapy since, in therapy, we are making him deal with the very thing he has been avoiding all of his life.

ESTABLISHING A CLINICAL VOCABULARY

To discuss the treatment of stuttering, we need to establish a clinical vocabulary. The following terms will be used throughout the book as we discuss stuttering therapy. The terminology that is unique to stuttering itself is presented and discussed in later chapters.

Clinical Vocabulary

Behavior. A behavior is anything a person does. Overt behaviors are actions or movements which can be observed. Covert behaviors are thoughts or feelings which can not be observed but are still considered behaviors. There is a concept known as the "dead man" rule which indicates that anything a living person can do that a dead man cannot do is a behavior. This should give us room to operate!

Behaviors have three characteristics which we will be concerned with: their frequency of occurrence, their strength or intensity when they occur, and their duration once they do occur. We will be manipulating these characteristics as we move through therapy.

Stimulus (S). This is anything that attracts a person's attention. It may be something inside the person, such as a headache, or something in the external environment, such as objects in a room. We will not view a stimulus as an event which "elicits" a behavior but rather as an event which prompts or cues a behavior to occur. The behavior may be either overt or covert.

Response (R). This is the reaction a person has to a stimulus, a behavior. Responses include thinking about the stimulus, looking at an object in a room, imitating a speech behavior presented by the clinician, rewarding a client for a correct behavior, and other such behaviors by either the client or the clinician.

Antecedent event. This is any event that precedes the response, that is, the stimulus that prompts or cues a response to occur.

Modeling. This is the demonstration of a behavior. We show the clients what we want them to do. This includes such diverse behaviors as the production of the [ɝ] sound, maintaining eye contact, opening the jaw further during speech, slowing down the rate of speech, using the correct syntax, and so forth. This is the demonstration of the *behavior change goal* so that our clients know what we expect them to do.

Information. In our contact with the client we can either provide for the client or request from the client two types of information. First, we can provide *behavioral* information that is concerned with the behavior we are attempting to teach. This type of information includes such things as telling the client to prolong the vowel when attempting to slow down the rate of speech, or to hold the teeth closer together when attempting to make the [s] sound. We can also request the client to repeat what we have said to him to make sure he understood us.

Second, we can provide *general* information. This includes a description of our therapy, the therapy goals, information to change attitudes or emotions, and so forth. Again, we might ask the client to repeat what we have told him to determine his perception of what we said.

Guidance. Another term for guidance would be "prompt." There are four types of guidance that we use in therapy. We give *verbal* guidance in the form of hints or cues about the performance of a behavior.

Gestural guidance would be those gestures we make to prompt or cue a behavior to occur. We also use *environmental* guidance when we manipulate the environment so that it elicits the behavior, for example, showing the client a picture. Finally, we use *physical* guidance when we actually touch the client to assist in the performance of a behavior.

Contingent event. This is any event that follows the response. Basically, this means either a pleasant event (reward) or an unpleasant event (penalty).

Reward (R +). This means the same as reinforcement. It signifies the positive event that occurs after a behavior is performed. If the event is truly rewarding to the client, the chances of the behavior occurring again are increased.

Penalty (P). This means the same as punishment. It signifies the negative event that occurs after a behavior is performed. If the event is truly penalizing to the client, the chances of the behavior occurring again are decreased.

Extinguish. When reward for a behavior is withheld, the behavior will extinguish. It will cease to occur since with no reward, the behavior no longer has a purpose. However, if the behavior has become self-rewarding it will continue to occur since it is no longer dependent on an external reward.

Reward schedule. When we use this term we are referring to how often we reward a behavior. A *continuous schedule* means that we reward every occurrence of a behavior. This provides fast learning but the behavior is not very stable and will have a tendency to cease when the reward is removed. With an *intermittent schedule* we reward on a more random basis. There are two types of intermittent systems, ratio and interval. In the ratio system, either fixed or variable, the reward is given based on the number of times the behavior has occurred. In the interval system, the determining factor for reward is time. The intermittent schedule is not as efficient for learning a behavior but makes the behavior very stable and the behavior will have a tendency to continue even after the reward is removed.

Approach motivation. This represents the mental attitude of the client where the focus of therapy is on rewards. He will perform the behavior being rewarded more often in order to get more rewards.

Avoidance motivation. This represents the mental attitude of the client where the focus of therapy is on penalties. He will perform the behavior being penalized less often in order to avoid the penalty.

Shaping. This is the process of creating a *new* behavior in a client. As behaviors more closely approximate the target behavior they are rewarded and through this process the new behavior is gradually "shaped."

Significant others. These are people who are very important in the client's life, usually the client's parents, foster parents, relative, wife, husband, or close friend.

Token economy. When the client is initially rewarded with tokens, such as poker chips, which he can turn in at some later time for a more meaningful reward, this is referred to as a *token economy.*

Stimulus control. Stimuli can be manipulated in several ways. They can be gradually presented, gradually withdrawn, increased in number, decreased in number, or their prompting role changed.

Fading. This is the gradual removal of a stimulus. We can gradually withdraw our model of a behavior. We are then fading the model. Also, when we give the client a reward, it is a stimulus for him. When we gradually withdraw the rewards, we are fading them.

THE CLINICIAN/CLIENT INTERACTION

The clinical interactions between the clinician and the client are presented here as a series of "transactions." We will illustrate the transaction by using some of the terms we have just defined. The initial communication between the clinician and the client would appear as:

$$S—O—R$$

The (S) represents the clinician presenting the initial stimulus; the (O) stands for "organism" and represents the client's cognition of the stimulus; and the (R) represents the client's response to the clinician after he has thought about what he should do. It is now the clinician's turn to respond to the client. The diagram is then expanded to:

$$S—O—R/S—O—R$$

The (S) in this part of the transaction now represents the client's response, (R), as it becomes the stimulus S for the clinician. The (O) represents the clinician's cognition of the stimulus; and the (R) represents the clinician's response to the client. This completes the first transaction. In her cognitions during the transaction the clinician must (1) evaluate the correctness of the response for either a reward or a penalty, (2) determine if the correct response is occurring more often, (3) evaluate the attentiveness of the client to the therapy, and (4) determine how to initiate the next transaction. The direction of the next transaction is dependent on how successful the current transaction has been. If the client's response was correct and the client was attending to therapy, she can proceed to the next step in therapy. If the response was not correct or the client was not attending to therapy, she will have to repeat this transaction or deal with the client's lack of attentiveness.

The type of response the clinician gives to the client is extremely important. If the response is a reward, she will be creating approach motivation in the client. However, if the response is a penalty, she will be creating avoidance motivation in the client. These forms of motivation are vital to successful therapy and are directly controlled by the clinician. Both motivational forms will be used in our therapy so it is important that you recognize their basic differences. With approach motivation the client is actively seeking the reward while with avoidance motivation the client is actively seeking to avoid the penalty.

There are *two* behavioral performances occurring in each transaction; the clinical behavior that the clinician is focusing on and the attending behavior of the client. Rewards and penalties will influence both forms of behavior. If attending behavior is rewarded, it will occur more often and, conversely, nonattending behavior will occur less often when it is penalized. In that the client must be attending to therapy if it is to be effective, the focus of therapy may occasionally shift to dealing with attending behaviors.

Having completed the first transaction, the clinician initiates the second transaction. This sequence then continues, with the direction of each transaction dependent on the preceding one. If you will, the transactions are like a string of beads; the clinician adds each bead to the string after the preceding one is in place. Another way to view the clinical transaction is in a circular mode as shown in Figure 2-1.

Each time the circle is completed it represents a clinical transaction. Consider the following example of two transactions with a stutterer.

S—Clinician demonstrates (models) a slow rate of speech.
O—Client perceives and thinks about the model.
R—Client speaks at a rate which he feels is like the model.
S—Client's speech is the stimulus for the clinician.
O—Clinician evaluates the client's speech.
R—Clinician says, "That was pretty good, but let's try it again"
　　　(penalty).

(End first transaction)

S—Clinician models the slow rate of speech again.
O—Client perceives and thinks about model.
R—Client speaks at a rate which he feels imitates the model.

S—Client's speech is the stimulus for the clinician.

O—Clinician evaluates the client's speech.

R—The clinician says, "That was very good, just like I did" (reward).

(End second transaction)

Transactional Testing

Each transaction represents the clinician's testing of how well the client is learning, his attending to therapy, and the effectiveness of the rewards and penalties. This testing is basic to therapy. It determines if a transaction must be repeated, if the focus of therapy must be shifted to attending behaviors, if the reward and/or the penalty must be changed, and how effective and efficient the therapy is. One of the most important aspects of testing concerns the effects the clinician's responses are having on the client, both in terms of the speech behavior and the attending behaviors. It is very important for the clinician to respond in some way to the client after each of his responses. The clinician may extinguish a new behavior by not responding to it. A behavior must have a reason to be performed, namely, a reward of some kind.

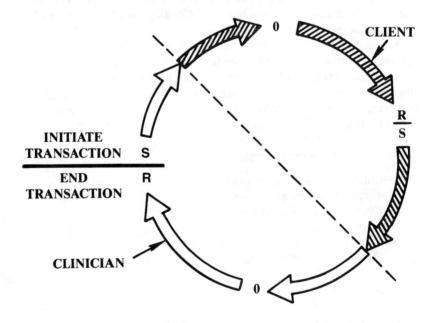

FIGURE 2-1

THE CLINICIAN'S TASKS

As indicated in the transactional diagram, the clinician has three specific tasks in each transaction. She must first of all provide the stimulus to start the transaction and prompt the client's response. Her next task is to evaluate the client's response and, finally, to respond to the client.

The Clinician's Stimulus (Starting the Transaction)

Modeling. Perhaps the most common form of stimulus used by the speech clinician is to "model" the behavior for the client. With stutterers we can model new speech behaviors that minimize the stuttering or model methods of dealing with stuttering blocks. When we speak of modeling, we are talking about the clinician demonstrating the behavior so that the client can attempt to imitate it. We are setting forth the behavior change goal for the client with the model. When he sees or hears it he knows what the clinician expects him to do.

Guidance. Guidance is leading or directing the client to the correct behavior or prompting it to occur. It can take the form of verbal, gestural, environmental, or physical guidance. An example of verbal guidance would be to say to the client, "Speak a bit slower, you are talking too fast." Verbal guidance (or verbal prompts) assist in the production of a behavior when the model is not present. Facial expressions and body or hand gestures are part of gestural guidance. Again, these are used to prompt a behavior or to modify it. If we gesture in such a way as to indicate that the stutterer should slow down his rate while he is speaking, this is gestural guidance. When we manipulate or change the clinical environment so that a desired behavior occurs, this is environmental guidance. An example of this would be to put the stutterer in a very comfortable chair to get him more relaxed so there will be less stuttering. If we should assist the relaxation by massaging the neck muscles of the stutterer, we would be adding physical guidance. The various forms of guidance can be used in any combination.

Information. There are two types of information. Behavioral information is information we give the client about how to produce the behavior he is attempting to perform. We might tell the stutterer that when he slows down the rate of speech, we want him to flow his words together and make the vowel sounds longer in duration. General information is that information we give our client that is related to therapy but not to the specific behavior. This would constitute such information as when the next therapy session will be, or giving him work to do at home.

We can also ask the client for information, such as asking him if he understands what we are telling him. We might have him repeat what we have said to see if he is paying attention. Other information we might want would concern his feelings about his stuttering when we are doing the initial evaluation of the stuttering.

The Clinician's Cognitions

The clinician must make some very important decisions after she hears and/or sees the client's responses. She is involved in evaluating the correctness of the response, determining if the correct response is occurring more often, evaluating the client's attentiveness to therapy, and deciding how she will start the next transaction.

The first three decisions determine if she moves ahead in therapy or if she must repeat the last transaction. This testing also tells her if she must shift her therapy from focusing on the speech to dealing with the client's attending behaviors and his approach or avoidance motivation.

With stuttering clients, the clinician must also be aware of the client's cognitive set: his attitudes, emotions, and feelings during the transactions. If any of these factors begin to negatively influence the treatment program, the clinician must deal with them. If these factors are positively influencing treatment, the clinician should take advantage of the opportunity to reward the positive cognitive set. In some instances where the negative influence is totally disrupting treatment, the focus of therapy may have to be shifted for a period of time while the clinician deals with the client's cognitive set. This is discussed further in chapter 5.

The Clinician's Responses (Ending the Transaction)

Reward. This is an event that occurs following the behavior that the client sees as a positive consequence. Through approach motivation, the client is motivated to get the reward by performing the behavior that is rewarded. Approach motivation is extremely important to therapy. However, in selecting something for a reward, we must remember that we can not determine if it is actually a reward until its effect on the client's behavior is studied. An event can only be labeled a "reward" if its presentation results in an increase in the frequency of occurrence of the behavior. Many clinicians decide on a "reward" by selecting things *they* feel are rewarding and then they never check to see what effect it is having on the client and his behavior. You may feel that a very chewy candy is a reward but if the client has braces on his teeth, this could be a penalty for the client. However, if therapy must wait until the candy is cleaned from the braces and your therapy is boring, the delay, not the candy, may be the reward for the client. Rewards must be selected with the client's likes and dislikes in mind. So, when we make a decision on what we are going to use as a reward, we must observe the effect that it has on the client and the behavior.

There are two types of rewards we can give our clients: primary rewards and secondary rewards. Primary rewards are directed to basic needs such as food and water. Secondary rewards are more social in nature and are learned. This includes such things as praise or giving the client a token as a reward. With either form of reward we must consider the strength and the timing of the reward, how appropriate it is for our clinical setting, and how often we present it.

The strength of the reward is dependent on how important it is to the client. If the reward has little value to the client, it is not a strong reward. However, if the reward is highly valued by the client, it is a strong reward. The stronger the reward, the higher the client's approach motivation; he will be highly motivated to get the reward. Further, if the clinician has good rapport with the client, any reward is strengthened since the clinician is an important person to the client and this makes the reward more significant.

The timing of the reward is crucial. There cannot be too long a period of time between the performance of the behavior and the receiving of the reward. The client must associate the performance of the specific behavior with the presentation of the reward. If another behavior occurs between the desired behavior and the presentation of the reward, it is the second behavior that is being rewarded since the reward is contingent to it.

The appropriateness of the reward must also be considered. Food is not an appropriate reward if the client is to consume it immediately after it is presented; as with our example of the chewy candy, this may take up the rest of the time scheduled for therapy. It would be better if the client had to wait until after therapy to consume it. The client would now have to get the candy out of his braces on his own time, not during your clinical time. More appropriate rewards would be verbal praise, stickers (stars, characters, science fiction), an ink stamp on the hand, additional recess or library time, transfers, plastic toys, or tokens.

Then there is also the schedule of presentation of the reward to consider. The two types of schedules are *continuous* and *intermittent*. With the continuous reward schedule, the reward is presented every time the behavior is performed, in other words, a ratio of 1:1. This leads to rapid learning but, when the reward is removed, rapid extinction; that is, the behavior disappears quickly when the reward is removed.

With the intermittent reward schedule we no longer reward every behavioral performance. We may reward every other performance (a 2:1 ratio) or every third performance (a 3:1 ratio). We can also reward more on a random basis. This type of schedule does not lend itself to rapid learning, but it does reduce the probability of extinction. The behavior tends to continue even after the reward has been removed since there is still a chance that a reward will be forthcoming. In therapy, we normally start out with a continuous reward schedule for fast learning and then shift to an intermittent schedule to resist extinction when the rewards are eliminated.

There are some people who object to the use of rewards in therapy. They feel that the client is being bribed to perform his new speech behavior, and the word "bribe" has negative connotations. If the reward is viewed as "payment" for work done, then we are able to avoid the bribe concept. This payment concept also gives us a means of explaining our clinical procedure to parents who might object to rewards from this standpoint, by drawing an analogy between his or her receiving a pay check for work they have accomplished and the reward their child receives for clinical "work" he has accomplished.

Penalty. Theoretically, if the incorrect productions of a speech behavior are ignored, that is, there is no contingent event, the behavior should extinguish. However, the speech behavior is usually strongly habituated and self-rewarding. A more efficient means of dealing with the incorrect speech productions is to penalize their occurrence in some way. Most clinicians respond to incorrect productions by saying to the client, "That was not very good" or "I think you can do that better." This is a form of penalty. Penalty does not have to be harsh or severe. When the client is informed that the production was not correct and this is interpreted by the client as a penalty, there will be a decrease in occurrence of the incorrect behavior. The client will develop avoidance motivation and will not perform the behavior that is penalized. Penalizing the behavior is a more efficient way to eliminate a behavior than relying on extinction to occur.

We must apply the same rules to a penalty that we applied to a reward. We must determine if our response is actually a penalty, determine the strength of the penalty, the contingency or timing of the penalty, and consider the appropriateness of the penalty. A response can be considered a penalty only if the frequency of occurrence of the penalized behavior decreases. The strength of the penalty must also be carefully considered as well as how often it is applied. As was stated earlier, the penalty need not be severe or harsh, just strong enough so that the client would prefer to avoid it. We must be careful not to apply too much penalty since this has a negative effect on the morale of the client. Also, when we apply penalty we should also be consistent in its application. Nothing is more disconcerting than to be penalized inconsistently for something we have done.

Finally, we must decide on a penalty that is appropriate not only to the client but also to the work environment. A clinician who levies a fine of one dollar for each occurrence of an incorrect response might make a lot of money early in therapy but would sooner or later face some problems with her administration. Public institutions such as the schools are sensitive to public opinion and the penalty you use should be carefully determined.

The two basic forms of penalty are penalty by administration, and by withdrawal. We can administer such penalties as requiring the client to repeat a behavior or giving him verbal penalty. Penalty by withdrawal would constitute the removal of a reward, such as the removal of a token or a distracting object. We can also remove the client from the clinical environment where he receives rewards. This does not necessarily mean having the client leave therapy and return to the classroom. With some therapy I have observed, this would be a reward for the client. If the client is in a group where he is receiving rewards and we remove him from the group, we have removed his opportunity to receive rewards. This is a form of "time out" and is a commonly used form of penalty. However, with either form of penalty we are still creating avoidance motivation as the client attempts to avoid the penalty by not performing the behavior.

Again, we will find people who object to the use of penalty with a client. The use of penalty in therapy creates more negative reactions than the use of reward. However, if we think carefully about all learning environments, penalty is a common feature. All parents use some form of penalty in raising their children. There are obvious exceptions where parents never penalize their children, regardless of their behavior, and most clinicians have a special name for these children. But, we must also recognize that all speech clinicians use some form of penalty in their therapy, even if no more than telling the client that he did not perform the behavior correctly. All people learn to avoid things through penalty. It is a valuable form of learning.

THE CLINICAL INTERACTION MODEL (CIM)

We will now combine the learning orientations with the clinician/client transactions to form a model of clinical interactions. The clinical interaction model (CIM) is presented in Figure 2-2. The basic (S—O—R/S—O—R) transaction has been expanded to include all of the clinician's and client's activities. It also illustrates the influence of the clinician's responses, either reward or penalty, on the client's approach/avoidance motivation and his attending behaviors. This model will serve as a clinical guide in your stuttering therapy. The model will also be of assistance in analyzing any problems you might have in therapy, such as the client not comprehending your model or information.

The key word associated with both the clinician's stimulus and her response is "appropriate." The judgment of appropriateness is a clinical judgment that only the clinician can make. However, she should be aware that, if an adjustment must be made in therapy, the adjustment should be made by the clinician in terms of her modifying her stimulus and/or her response. For example, if the clinician presents the client with information that is too complex, beyond the cognitive level of the client, constant repetition of the information will accomplish nothing except to frustrate the client. To get the client to comprehend the information, the clinician must adjust it to the cognitive level of the client. This might mean rephrasing the information and/or changing the terminology used. Further, if the clinician is requesting a behavioral performance that is beyond the ability of the client, we again create frustration in the client. The clinician must recognize that her behavioral request was not appropriate for the functional level of the client. The stimulus from the clinician must be appropriate for the individual client.

The concept of "appropriateness" also applies to the clinician's rewards and penalties. As was stated earlier, they must be appropriate for the client and for the work environment. And the client is the only one who can determine if the clinician's response is a reward or penalty. A reward or penalty is not appropriate if the client does not interpret them as such. There are also rewards and penalties that are not appropriate for various clinical environments. The clinician must make this judgment as she assesses her work environment.

Finally, the CIM also demonstrates the relationship between the speech behavior and the attending behavior of the client. Appropriate rewards and penalties will maintain the client's approach and avoidance motivation and this fosters the attending behavior. However, if the client loses his motivation he will not be attending to therapy. In this instance the clinician must shift her clinical focus from the speech behavior to attending behavior since the client will not learn if he is not paying attention. The clinician must reevaluate her reward and penalty and modify them if they have lost their effect. Having done this, she could reward the client's attending behavior or penalize the nonattending behavior as she tells a story. She will have temporarily shifted therapy

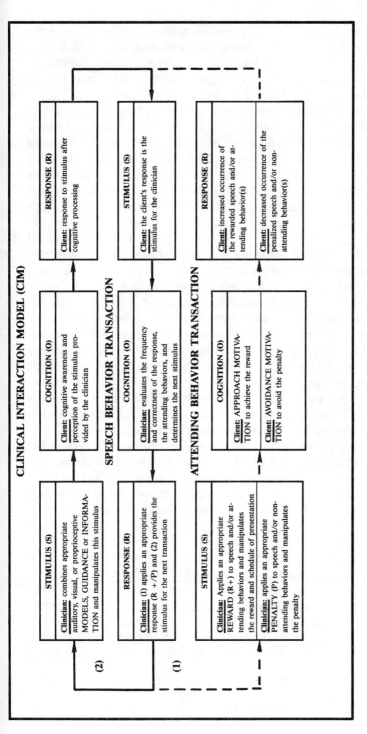

FIGURE 2-2

Clinical Interaction Model (CIM). Clinical Interaction Model (CIM) illustrates the two clinical transactions that are occurring simultaneously in therapy. The clinician is attending to the speech behaviors of the client as well as his attending behaviors. The focal point of therapy is the speech behavior, but, if the attending behavior becomes a problem, she can focus her therapy on the client's motivation and attending behaviors. Her response to the client, either reward or penalty, is very critical. It not only affects the occurrences of the client's speech behaviors, it also influences the client's motivation in therapy.

from the speech behavior to attending behavior. However, once the client's attention and motivation are reestablished, she can shift back to the speech behavior, making sure she does not loose the client's attention as she does so. This is a vital aspect of the CIM since all therapy is dependent on the client's attending to the clinician.

Before we leave the discussion of the CIM, let us go through it step by step. The clinical interaction begins with the clinician's stimulus, which is a combination of the factors listed in the CIM. The next step is the client's cognition or thinking about the stimulus. After thinking about the stimulus the client responds. This response is the stimulus for the clinician and she then thinks about and evaluates the response in terms of the frequency and correctness of the response, the client's attention to therapy, and how to start the next transaction. When her evaluation is completed, she responds to the client with either a reward or penalty. The next transaction is now ready to begin. However, the clinician's reward or penalty also has an effect on the client's attending behaviors, his motivation. Rewards increase the approach motivation while penalties increase the avoidance motivation. These then have the effect of increasing the occurrences of attending behaviors and the speech behavior (rewards) or decreasing the occurrences of nonattending behaviors or the incorrect speech behavior (penalty). During therapy the clinician focuses on the speech behavior transactions while monitoring the client's motivation and attending behavior. If there is a problem with motivation and attention, she shifts her focus to these areas until she again has the client's attention and motivation. She can then shift therapy back to the speech behaviors.

The CIM represents all of your clinical interactions. It applies not only to your client, but to all interactions where you are attempting to teach a new concept, belief, or behavior or where you are gathering information, such as during an interview or an evaluation. You will use the CIM in a teaching mode with your client, his parents, and his teachers. If you have a home program for a client you will have to teach the parents how to carry on the program. You will also teach the classroom teacher how to respond to the client if you involve her in the program. The information-gathering mode will also be used with the client, the parents, and the teacher as you monitor your program's success in the home and other speech environments. The CIM is the core of all clinical transactions.

The answers to the word puzzles earlier in the chapter? See if you can find the following: stuttering block, defect in speech, and break in eye contact.

Chapter 3

Special Clinical Operant Procedures

STIMULUS CONTROL

Manipulation of the stimulus is known as *stimulus control*. This is an important feature in all phases of therapy but especially important as we generalize the new speech behavior to other environments. Our stuttering clients have become conditioned to respond in certain ways to various stimuli in their environments and these "conditioned" stimuli are a very important factor in our stuttering therapy. In this book, we view the stimulus as anything in the environment that attracts the attention of the client and causes him to react in some way.

Thus far we have limited our discussion of the stimulus to that which is provided by the clinician. We will now broaden our view to include other forms of stimuli which influence the client. More specifically, we will consider three types of stimuli: the people the stutterer talks to such as his teacher, the speaking situations the stutterer encounters, like reciting in class, and objects the stutterer associates with speaking, like the telephone.

Conditioned Stimuli

Stimuli that are consistently associated with reward or penalty become conditioned so that they "cue" the stutterer as to what the outcome will be if a particular behavior is performed. Conditioned stimuli are referred to as *discriminative stimuli*. They do not *elicit* a behavioral response but rather prompt or cue the behavior to occur or to be avoided. Since the individual "knows" what the outcome will be if he performs the behavior, he has some influence over whether or not the behavior occurs. Positive cues will encourage the performance of a response while negative cues will discourage the performance of a response. Thus, the stimulus cues have a direct influence on the probability of the behavior occurring.

Positive stimuli. These are stimuli which have been conditioned to a positive outcome, a reward. They will be referred to as *positive stimuli*, or *S+* in the book. An ice cream cone on a hot day has become an S+ to most of us. The ice cream cone signifies that if we eat it, the experience will be rewarding. The ice cream cone was not originally a conditioned stimulus. It became a conditioned S+ only after we had eaten some on a hot day and found it rewarding. An association was then made between the ice cream cone and the reward of eating it.

In that rewards are associated with therapy, stimuli in that environment quickly assume the role of S+. When a speech behavior is rewarded and the reward is associated with the clinician, she becomes an S+. Thus, when she is present, the client is cued that if the specific speech behavior is performed, he will be rewarded. Even the clinic room becomes an S+ role, cuing the occurrence of the behavior that is rewarded.

Negative stimuli. Stimuli associated with a negative outcome, a penalty, assume the role of *negative stimuli* or *S-*. There are many such cues in our lives. S- cues, for example, influence the way we drive our cars. Let us say that we are driving our car a bit over the posted speed limit when a police car, an S-, is sighted. We quickly reduce our speed to the posted limit so as to avoid receiving a speeding ticket, a rather severe penalty. We know that driving too fast results in a traffic ticket, so we avoid the ticket by not performing the behavior. What happens to the speed of our car when the patrol car is out of sight is left to your imagination. Signs also serve as S- cues. This would include signs such as "keep out," "do not enter," "beware of the dog," "wrong way," "do not touch," and "if it breaks, you bought it." Doors with signs "men" or "women" on them can also assume an S- role, especially when we have just entered the wrong one.

If the client performs a behavior and the clinician consistently responds by penalizing him, she assumes the role of S- for that behavior. The behavior may be a disruptive behavior such as wandering around the clinic room, nonattending behavior in the form of looking out the window, or an incorrect speech behavior. The S- role is important, not only in direct therapy, but also in establishing control over clients whose behaviors interfere with therapy.

If the client avoids the penalty by not performing the negative behavior, what behavior does he perform? He will search for a behavior that will not be penalized or, if we have taught him an alternate behavior, he will perform it, especially if it results in a reward. So, by performing the behavior we have taught him, he can not only avoid the penalty but also achieve the reward. For example, a client who stutters is talking to us and his rate of speech increases. He immediately senses that he will be penalized by the clinician (S-) for the fast rate. But he also recognizes the clinician as an S+ for a slower rate. So, he shifts to a slower rate of speech. By doing this he not only avoids the penalty (a form of negative reward) but also gets a direct reward. Thus, the slower rate of speech is rewarded twice.

The effects of penalty are complex. They do not extinguish a behavior, but they do reduce its frequency of occurrence. However, in that we are dealing with clients who stutter, the effects of penalty have some other ramifications, such as increased tension or anxiety. This does not mean that we do not use penalty with the stutterer. It only means that we must understand what the ramifications are and apply penalty accordingly. Most important of all: *we do not penalize a behavior until the client has an alternative behavior he can perform to avoid the penalty.*

Neutral stimuli. In addition to the stimulus roles of S+, prompting the correct production of the speech behavior, and S-, prompting the avoidance of the penalty by not producing the incorrect behavior, the clinician can assume a third stimulus role. This is the role of *neutral stimuli* or *S0*. This stimulus cues that there will be no consequence for the behavior. If a behavior is not rewarded (or rewarding), it has no purpose, no reason to exist. When this situation exists, the behavior extinguishes.

Stimulus Manipulation

The clinician is able to manipulate these stimuli in a number of ways. These manipulations are very important to our stuttering therapy. The five forms of stimulus manipulation will be discussed individually.

Shifting the role of the stimuli. A stimulus may have been conditioned to an S+, S-, or S0 role but these roles can be changed. If the parents penalized the client for his stuttering, their role is an S-. However, if they are counseled so that they no longer penalize the stuttering, their role will shift to S0. Or, if the parents reward the stuttering in the home, they are an S+, maintaining the stuttering in the home environment. Their S+ role can be shifted to an S0 by removing the reward. We can change the stimulus role by associating the stimulus with a different contingent event. This will be an important factor if we are able to establish a home program to supplement our work in the clinical environment. This is especially important as we generalize the new speech to environments outside the clinic room.

A rule of thumb in shifting stimulus roles is that any stimulus, regardless of its current role, when consistently associated with reward, becomes an S+. When associated with penalty, stimuli become S- and when there is no contingent event, the stimuli become S0.

Gradual introduction of stimuli. If an S- is too threatening and overwhelms the client, we may find that we must introduce the S- gradually, allowing the client time to adjust to it. A client who stutters may find it extremely frightening to speak in front of a group. When he is in front of a group, he is so frightened that he can not use his new speech behavior. We can gradually introduce this S- situation by starting with one listener. When the client can perform satisfactorily with one listener and the situation becomes an S+, we can then add another listener. This process is repeated. We are gradually introducing the stimuli while keeping the situation at an emotional level where the client can perform his new speech behavior. The speaking situation gradually then shifts from an S- to an S+ (or at least to a very weak S-) as he learns that he can speak in front of a group. In this example we are gradually increasing the strength or intensity of the stimulus. We can also manipulate the frequency and the duration of stimuli in this way if the need arises.

Gradual withdrawal of stimuli. The stimulus can also be gradually withdrawn or faded. We do this by presenting it less often (frequency), in a weaker form (strength or intensity), or for a shorter period of time (duration). We can fade the model as the client learns the new speech behavior or we can fade the influence of our S+ role by not rewarding as much. Fading makes the new speech behavior more independent. We must eventually fade all stimuli so that the new speech behavior is being performed independent of prompts or cues.

Increase the number of stimuli. We must increase the number of S+ in the client's speaking environments if we are to achieve carry-over of the new speech behavior. These S+ will cue the new speech behavior to occur in other environments such as in the school, the home, on the job, and so forth. This form of manipulation is dependent on the client's significant others or cooperative people in the environment. However, as will be pointed out later, we can also create S+ by using inanimate objects. This form of stimulus manipulation is extremely important. The efficiency of our therapy in terms of generalizing the new speech to other speaking environments is dependent upon the number of S+ in the client's life.

Decrease the number of stimuli. We may also find the need to reduce the number of stimuli in the client's clinical environment. The stuttering client may be overwhelmed by the number of other clients in a group or other distractions in the clinical room. If the client can not function in a large group, he might be placed in a smaller group or even given individual therapy until he can handle a small group (gradual introduction of stimuli). If he is distressed by an object in the room, perhaps it can be removed. To many stutterers, a tape recorder is an S- and its presence in the clinic room might interfere with therapy.

PROCEDURES FOR DELIVERY OF REWARDS AND PENALTIES

There are special procedures that we will use as we present rewards and/or penalties. The first procedure, *shaping,* concerns itself with what behaviors receive rewards while the second procedure, the *token economy,* addresses the issue of what is used as a reward. The procedures can be used independently or they can be combined. In other words, a clinician can use a token economy with the shaping procedure.

Shaping

Shaping is used to create new behaviors in the client. It is an operant technique where, in its purest form, the goal behavior is not identified for the client. Thus, the behaviors that do occur are not goal oriented but, rather, more random in nature. Behaviors that approximate the goal behavior are rewarded while all other behaviors are ignored. The reward increases the probability that goal-oriented behaviors will occur again. Behaviors that are not rewarded extinguish. The criteria for reward are steadily increased so that the goal behavior is eventually the only behavior that will be rewarded. This process is known as "successive approximation."

A form of shaping has been used for years by the speech clinician. However, when the speech clinician uses shaping, she improves the efficiency of the process by providing the client with the goal behavior through modeling, guidance, and information. Since the client then knows what the goal behavior is, all of his behavioral attempts are goal oriented. She also supplements the operant conditioning with cognitive learning through guidance and information she provides for the client. The most important aspect of this process is that it recognizes that most learning occurs in gradual steps, not "all at once."

Token Economy

The token economy is a unique procedure for administering rewards (or penalties) to a client. A major problem faced when giving a specific reward to a client is that, over time, the client becomes "bored" or satiated with the reward. A different type of problem faces the clinician in group therapy. She has a difficult time finding a single reward that is appropriate for all group members. The token economy solves both of these problems.

The client (or clients) are given "tokens" as rewards. Tokens can be anything that the clinician identifies as having "purchasing power." A common form of token is a poker chip. The clients accumulate tokens they receive as rewards during therapy time and then redeem them for a tangible reward, a "backup reward," after the therapy session is finished. The tokens themselves become rewarding after the client realizes that they will purchase a backup reward.

When using the token economy, the clinician has a great deal of flexibility in terms of her rewards. The token economy allows her to select a variety of items to use as backup rewards. This means that each client can choose his own reward. The clinician can also set "prices" for the rewards. If a client wants an "expensive" reward, he will have greater approach motivation to get tokens so he can purchase the item.

The clinician may also include a penalty in the token economy, withdrawing a token if a behavior is performed incorrectly. She can use this to create avoidance motivation. The client will avoid performing the behavior incorrectly to prevent the clinician from removing a token. In this situation the clinician has created both approach and avoidance motivation in the client. This will be a very effective and efficient therapy procedure.

The token reward schedule should change as the behavior becomes more firmly established. The reward schedule would shift from continuous reward to intermittent reward. This will strengthen the behavior and make it more resistant to extinction as the reward is removed. It is wise to pair the token with verbal praise. When the token economy is terminated, the praise can be used, if necessary, to maintain the behavior until it becomes self-rewarding.

Some advantages of token rewards over traditional rewards are the providing of a variety of rewards, not interrupting therapy while the client "consumes" a reward, making it easier to administer the reward, and giving the same initial reward to all clients in a group setting. The token economy is an extremely useful clinical tool for the speech clinician. It will be used extensively in the stuttering therapy program presented in this book.

We must also consider the effectiveness of the token economy with older clients. The clinician faces problems in that the token economy calls for cooperation on the part of the client. Some older clients may feel that the procedure is childish and will not cooperate. There is little the clinician can do in this instance. However, if the client (or clients) are willing to cooperate, the clinician must then find some backup reward that is important for each client. This is more difficult with older clients but can be done with some imagination and client input.

Chapter 4

Behavioral Aspects of Stutterers

AN OPERATIONAL DESCRIPTION OF STUTTERING

We start our discussion of stuttering by considering the behavioral aspects, since it is the stuttering itself which is the basis of the negative cognitive set of the stutterer. Once we have considered the behaviors associated with stuttering we can better understand the stutterer's cognitive reaction to it.

First, an operational description of stuttering. We can work from this base as we examine the behaviors that constitute what we refer to as stuttering. The disorder of stuttering is not a single behavioral event but is made up of a combination of interrelated behaviors. Stuttering consists of repetitions and/or prolongations of sounds, syllables, and words, but this is true only in that all individuals who stutter have repetitions and/or prolongations. The phenomenon of stuttering is much more complex. In addition to the repetitions and prolongations, we find other behaviors that the stutterer uses to terminate or avoid the repetitions and prolongations. These behaviors are referred to as secondary mannerisms, accessory features, or anxiety-reducing behaviors. Because stuttering is so complex and comprises so many behavioral events, we face many problems when we attempt to assess the "severity" of the stuttering. To complicate the assessment even more, we must consider four characteristics of each behavior, that is, how often or frequently it occurs, how strong or intense it is when it occurs, its duration once it occurs, and its appropriateness when it occurs.
occurs.

Severity Scales as Describers

When we use a formal (standardized) or informal (not standardized) scale to assess the severity of stuttering we consider all of these points. The formal scale that is recommended is the Stuttering Severity Index by Riley (1972). This scale takes into consideration not only the frequency and duration of stuttering blocks, but also the degree of "distraction" associated with the secondary mannerisms. The reference cited above includes not only all of the information concerning standardization of the scale but also a copy of the form used.

Informal scales are those severity scales which are created by various clinical programs to be used by the speech clinicians in that program. They are also concerned with the frequency, intensity, and duration of behaviors associated with stuttering but they are somewhat limited in their use. They are of value within the program since all of the clinicians understand the form and how to use it. However, if the information is transmitted to another clinical program there may be a great deal of confusion as to the definitions of terms and the means of judging the stuttering.

With almost all formal or informal scales of severity we are involved in counting the number of "blocks," the occurrences of repetitions and prolongations. We are concerned here with the frequency with which they occur. We also become involved in measuring the duration of the stuttering blocks. The strength or intensity of the block is also measured but indirectly through the amount of struggle behavior (secondary mannerisms) that is associated with the block. We consider the appropriateness of the block when we differentiate between "normal dysfluencies" and "stuttering blocks."

The same criteria are used when we examine the secondary mannerisms. We attempt to determine how often each behavior occurs. It is important to recognize that some behaviors occur too often while others may not occur often enough. In other words, we can have too little eye contact or too much. With too little eye contact, the stutterer never looks at his listener, looking everywhere but where he should. On the other hand, stutterers who have worked with clinicians who insist on unyielding eye contact often resemble a mongoose when attacking a cobra—never breaking eye contact, staring a hole through the listener. This behavior is more appropriate for hypnosis than friendly social interactions. We are also involved in some form of estimation of the strength or intensity of the mannerism when it occurs as well as its duration. The factor of appropriateness of a mannerism is quite difficult to assess since mannerisms are made up of normally occurring behaviors and it is often impossible to determine if the behavior was occurring normally or functioning as a mannerism.

All of this may be a bit vague, so let us consider the eye blink as a mannerism. We need to determine if the stutterer uses too many eye blinks or too few. In one instance the eyes are constantly blinking and this is distracting to the listener. On the other hand, the stutterer may "never" blink his eyes and this can be distracting as well. We are also concerned about the intensity of the eye blinks as they occur. If the eye blink is very hard, causing the eyebrow to wrinkle, this is an intense behavior which distracts the listener. When we consider the duration aspect, we must look at either the individual eye blink or, if the eye blinks occur in a rapid series where each eye blink is directly associated with the next, the series of eye blinks. With the individual eye blink, if the duration is too long the blink turns into an eye closure. If the eye blink occurs and the eyes "flutter" with eight or nine blinks occurring as a chain of behaviors, we must consider the duration of the chained event. We will have a problem when we attempt to determine the appropriateness of the eye blink. There will be many occasions when we can directly associate the eye blink with the stuttering block and there are other occasions when we know the eye blink was a normal function. But there are many times when we cannot determine with any accuracy which function the eye blink is serving.

With all of these behaviors involved and with four different factorial judgments to make, is it any wonder that we have difficulty in establishing the severity of stuttering? Behavioral analyses are difficult enough with single behaviors, let alone a phenomenon that is made up of numerous interrelated behaviors. As can be seen, stuttering is a complex behavioral event.

BEHAVIORS ASSOCIATED WITH STUTTERING

As has been demonstrated, stuttering is not a single behavioral event but is actually made up of many interrelated behaviors. Essentially, the behaviors can be classified in two categories, stuttering behaviors and associated or related behaviors, that is, secondary mannerisms.

Stuttering Behaviors

Stuttering behaviors may be viewed as the only behaviors that all stutterers have in common, that is, stutterers have both repetitions and prolongations. These behaviors are stuttering. They represent the stuttering "block" that the stutterer is attempting to terminate or avoid.

Repetition. We will consider the repetition as an inappropriate repeating of an articulatory movement which impedes the forward movement of speech. The repetitions may or may not be rhythmic, depending on the amount of struggle behavior associated with them. In that they prevent speech from progressing, they are referred to as a stuttering "block."

Prolongations. The prolongation is an inappropriate prolonging of an articulatory position that impedes the forward movement of speech. The prolongation may be voiced or silent, and may bear no relationship to the sound the stutterer is attempting to produce. There is also struggle associated with the prolongation. Since prolongations also prevent speech from progressing, they are another form of the stuttering "block."

Secondary Mannerisms

The secondary mannerism represents the attempt on the part of the stutterer to avoid or terminate the stuttering block. It is a symptom of his fear of stuttering. The mannerism, as such, never occurs unless it is associated with a stuttering block, either in anticipation of an occurrence or during a block itself.

To review the process, when the stutterer finds himself in a block, he struggles in an attempt to release the word he is trying to say and in his struggle, a behavior occurs that does indeed terminate the block. This behavior is rewarded by the release of the block and elimination of the anxiety and fear. Since it was rewarded, the probability that this behavior will occur again is increased. The behavior becomes associated with the block, occurring each time the stutterer has a block. The stutterer then introduces the behavior before feared words so that he will not stutter on them. This new strategy is also successful. In this way, the stutterer uses the behavior both to avoid and to terminate blocks. However, over a period of time, the behavior loses most of its ability to avoid or terminate the block. So, the stutterer develops another behavior that will release the block, but he does not stop using the first behavior. Soon, the new behavior also loses most of its ability to avoid or terminate the block, so another behavior is adopted but, again, the former behavior is not given up.

As each successive behavior is adopted and then loses its effectiveness, there is an increasing number of behaviors that are associated with the block, making it an extremely complicated series of interrelated behaviors. Thus, what the listener is observing and hearing is not only the actual stuttering in the form of repetitions and prolongations, but also all of the mannerisms the stutterer has adopted. The mannerisms take one of two basic forms: verbal and nonverbal.

Verbal Mannerisms

The verbal mannerisms are behaviors that are directly related to the speech. These would include the following:

Language modifiers. Sounds, words, or phrases the stutterer uses to avoid the block are referred to as language modifiers. The stutterer may use the sound (uh) before a feared word to avoid stuttering. He would say, "uhMy name is Ken." When using a word to avoid stuttering, the stutterer might say, "Well, my name is Ken." A phrase could be used as follows, "Let me see, my name is Ken." The stutterer can adopt any sound, word, or phrase to be used in this manner.

Retrials. These are words or phrases repeated inappropriately to avoid stuttering. The stutterer will repeat the word or phrase until he feels that he will be able to say the word he fears. The stutterer would use a retrial as, "My name is—my name is—my name is Ken." Any word or phrase can be used as a retrial.

Rate of speech. Most stutterers speak at a rate that, for them, is too fast. Their speech mechanisms and/or language planning skills are not sufficient to carry the fast rate without the speech system breaking down. They speak very fast in order to "get the words out before they stutter" or to get the speech over with as soon as possible.

Postponement. When the stutterer uses postponement, he does not speak until he feels he can do so without stuttering. If he is asked a question, he may pretend to think about it until he feels he can answer without stuttering.

Nonverbal Mannerisms

These behavioral mannerisms are not directly related to the speech. They are general motor movements that occur in the body for a variety of reasons.

Eye gestures. The term "eye gestures" includes eye blinks, eye closures, eye movements, eye contact, or any other mannerism involving the eyes that the stutterer uses to avoid or terminate the stuttering block. These gestures often include behaviors such as frowning or squinting.

Tongue movements. Tongue movements include such things as tongue protrusion, tongue clicks or smacks, or other such inappropriate tongue movements used to modify the block.

Mouth movements. Pursing of the lips, opening the mouth very wide, and other such inappropriate mouth movements are included in this classification.

Head movements. When the head is nodded, jerked upward or downward, or turned in any direction in order to influence the stuttering, the movement is a nonverbal mannerism.

Body movements. Nonverbal mannerisms in this category include such things as arm swings, foot movements, finger or foot tapping, or gross body movements. Any body movement can be used as a nonverbal mannerism.

Breathing patterns. The stutterer may take in a deep breath in order to avoid or terminate a block. This may develop further into gasping or other breathing irregularities that the stutterer uses as a nonverbal mannerism.

THE DEVELOPMENT OF STUTTERING

We will not attempt to get into the theory of why the first repetitions and/or prolongations occur. Rather we will start with a dysfluent child who will eventually become a stutterer and trace the development of stuttering. We will view the early repetitions and prolongations as normal dysfluencies. At this stage the child is unaware of their existence and has no reaction when they occur. However, in some way, they are brought to his attention and the child becomes aware of the repetitions and prolongations. When he is attempting to say a word and the repetition occurs, the child becomes frustrated. He knows what he wants to say but the word will not "come out." This is a form of penalty and penalty results in searching behavior, searching for a way to escape from the penalty. In his searching for an escape, he introduces other behaviors and finally finds one, for example, the eye blink, that terminates the repetition. Now, whenever a repetition or prolongation occurs, he blinks his eyes and it is terminated. The eye blink is being strongly rewarded (negative reward) in that it removes the penalty. This means that the eye blink will occur more often; it is becoming a learned behavior, an automatic behavior. In that the eye blink is successful in terminating the block, the stutterer then starts to introduce the eye blink before he says words that he is beginning to fear. Again, the behavior is successful and is rewarded in that it avoids the block and allows the word to be spoken.

Unfortunately, the effectiveness of the eye blink soon weakens and no longer effectively avoids or terminates the dysfluency. Thus, more dysfluencies are occurring and they are lasting longer. The penalty of the dysfluency increases and the child starts to search for another means of escaping. This time he finds that if he stomps his foot the dysfluency is terminated. This new behavior is thus rewarded and becomes a learned, automatic behavior. However, the eye blink continues to occur, now along with the foot stamp. The eye blink continues to occur because it still occasionally avoids or terminates a dysfluency. This is intermittent reward which was discussed earlier as a strong form of learning which counteracts extinction. So now we have the child blinking his eyes and stomping his foot when dysfluencies occur. His frustration is growing and he is beginning to have doubts about his ability to escape from the dysfluencies. This is the beginning of the fear and anxiety associated with talking. Somewhere in this development, and we are not sure where, the child changes from a normally dysfluent speaker to a stutterer, even though the stuttering may be very mild.

Once the child associates fear and anxiety with talking and begins to struggle with the dysfluencies, he is a stutterer, the severity of which is not a factor. The dysfluencies are now stuttering blocks and the release behaviors he was using become secondary mannerisms. He is now on his way, developing the stuttering into more severe and complex forms. He will continue to add additional mannerisms as each previous one loses its effectiveness. Each mannerism continues to be associated with the stuttering block, making the blocks more complex.

The developmental process appears to continue through the late teens with the stutterer adding new fears and new mannerisms. Somewhere during the late teens, the stutterer seems to settle on a series of established mannerisms and no longer develops new ones. However, new fears continue to be established as he encounters new speaking situations and expands his social contacts. As will be noted in the following chapter, the emotional "development" of the stutterer regarding his reaction to his stuttering appears to also stop during the teen years. Perhaps it is at this time that the stutterer develops the belief that there is nothing that he can do about the stuttering. He develops a feeling of being a victim of the stuttering, helpless to do anything about it. This may explain why he no longer develops new mannerisms in an attempt to escape from the stuttering.

WHERE STUTTERING OCCURS

Now that we have some idea of what stuttering is, what behaviors are involved in the stuttering act, and how it develops, we should address the issues of where it occurs. This is a broad issue. It can be viewed from many angles but we limit our discussion to four aspects which are relevant to our therapy.

Physiologically

The repetition or prolongation can occur anywhere in the vocal tract where there is a point of articulation, that is, where two parts of the vocal tract come together during speech. For example, they can occur at the level of the vocal folds or at the lips. With the vocal folds, we are involved in openings and closings as required for speech, just as we are with the lips. However, with the vocal fold movements we are adjusting voicing while with the lips we are producing a phoneme. We can use a phonetic classification system of bilabial, lingual–alveolar, lingual–palatal, and so forth, to indicate where the stuttering block may occur, but we would have to add a category of glottal to account for the blocks that occur in the larynx. It is important to recognize that the blocks are not equally distributed among the points of articulation. There appear to be more bilabial, lingual–alveolar, and in other categories (DeVreugd, 1982).

Phonetically

The block does not occur on the phoneme itself, but rather, in the movement of the articulators from one position to the next. The stutterer may attempt to say his name, Peter, but will stutter by exhaling with his mouth open. He is not even getting his mouth into the position to say the (p) sound. He may even use vocalization in this example, which would result in his saying, "Uh----Peter." He is still not getting his articulators into the (p) position. Using the same example, the stutterer now says, "P------eter". He has his articulators in the correct position for the (p) but now is not moving them into the following vowel sound. He has correctly made the (p) but has not completed it since he must move into the vowel in order for the sound to be completed. Finally, our stutterer says his name by stuttering, "Puh—puh—puh—peter." He is not having any trouble saying the (p) sound; he made it four times. He is not moving his articulators from the (p) into the next sound. It is important to note that when he repeated the (p) sound, he did not move into the (e) sound as he should have but produced the (uh) sound, the schwa vowel, even though there is not schwa vowel in the word "Peter." It appears that the stutterer was trying to say the letter (P) rather than the word "Peter." If you ask the stutterer the sound of the letter (P), he will say "Puh" using the schwa vowel, just as he did when he stuttered on his name.

Linguistically

From this standpoint, almost all stuttering occurs when the stutterer initiates speech, when he starts to talk. We know that stutterers fragment their speech, that is, they stop and restart their speech on numerous occasions. This leads to a higher probability that they will stutter. If the stutterer says, "I have—to go—to my—math class—now," he has started speaking five times, once for each short phrase. His probability of stuttering is quite high. However, if he had eliminated the pauses and the restarting of his speech by saying, "I have to go to my math class now," he would reduce the probability of stuttering to a fifth of that for the first sentence.

Socially

Stuttering only occurs in a social environment. If the stutterer is alone, out of social contact, he will not stutter when he talks. However, when he is in a social environment, he is subjected to four general sources of communication stress. The first is the degree of propositionality of his speech: how much thinking and talking he must do, how abstract the message is that he is attempting to communicate. The more he has to think and talk at the same time, the more stress he is under and the more he will stutter. This aspect of communication stress is illustrated in the following examples.

> *Example 1:* The stutterer is looking at a picture and telling a story about what is happening in the picture. He must integrate all of the things happening in the picture and put them in a story, which he must make up at that instant.

> *Example 2:* The stutterer has been asked by another child his age how to put the chain back on a 10-speed bicycle. The bicycle is not present so the stutterer must describe the procedure very carefully.

The second factor is the listener. This includes who the listener is (a figure of authority, a peer, a person of the opposite sex), and how many listeners there are. This factor is present in the following examples.

> *Example 1:* The teacher has sent the stutterer to the principal to ask for something for the class. The stutterer must go into the principal's office and ask a specific question. The principal is a figure of authority for the stutterer.

> *Example 2:* The stutterer has written a very good paper for his class assignment and is asked to read it in front of the class. He has to read his paper in front of 20 peers and the teacher.

The next factor is the emotional content of what he is talking about. This can be either a positive or negative emotion, as is demonstrated in these examples.

> *Example 1:* The stutterer has broken a window while playing at home and must tell his parents that he broke it.

> *Example 2:* The stutterer found a $20 bill when coming home from school and he wants to tell his best friend about it.

The final source of communication stress is speaking while under time pressure. Rapid speech may be an actual requirement in the speaking situation or it may be only the stutterer's feeling that rapid speech is a requirement. Examples of this follow:

> *Example 1:* The classroom teacher is having her class respond quickly to questions in order to test their knowledge of a subject. She explains that each student must respond as quickly as possible to her questions.

> *Example 2:* The stutterer is standing in line at a fast food outlet. When it is his turn to order the person at the counter asks what he would like to order. There are many people waiting to order, so the person speaks very rapidly to the stutterer.

These sources of communication stress can occur individually, but in most speaking situations you will find more than one factor operating. In the following examples you will find that a variety of factors are involved in each situation.

> *Example 1:* The stutterer has broken some very serious rules in the school and has been asked to explain to a faculty committee why the rules were made and why he broke them.

> *Example 2:* After taking his date to a very nice restaurant for dinner, the stutterer finds that he left his wallet at home. He must explain this to the waiter as his date listens.

There is one other source of communication stress that is unique: the telephone. Almost all stutterers have some negative reaction to either calling on or answering the telephone. With the telephone, there is no direct contact between the stutterer and his listener except through the speech and this puts special demands on the speech production. There is also the problem of time pressure. When the telephone rings and the stutterer picks it up, he feels he must answer quickly. Or, if he calls someone and they answer, he feels he must respond quickly. If the stutterer has a long silent block on either calling or answering, the other party might well hang up the phone. This puts a lot of pressure on the stutterer to speak quickly. And, the more time pressure the stutterer puts on himself, the higher the probability that he will stutter.

TECHNIQUES TO MODIFY STUTTERING BEHAVIORS

Behaviors to Eliminate Stuttering

The approach we will be using in our therapy to modify stuttering is operant conditioning. As was discussed in an earlier chapter, behaviors that are rewarded tend to occur more often while behaviors that are penalized tend to occur less often. This is the basis of the behavioral aspect of our therapy. However, it is important to note that our program is not "fluency" oriented, that is, we are not rewarding fluent speech. *We reward the new speech behavior which, when performed, results in controlled fluency.* The term *new speech behavior* is used to describe the new way we will teach the client to speak. Actually, we will be changing four aspects of speech to achieve the new speech behavior. The four aspects we will be changing are (1) slower *rate* of speech; (2) attending to oral cues or *enunciation;* (3) *easy onset* of vocalization, and (4) smooth *flow* of speech, together referred to as REEF. When the client performs his REEF, he is performing his new speech behavior, which results in controlled fluency. These aspects of speech are modified simultaneously rather than one at a time. In other words, the new speech behavior is viewed as a behavior in and of itself. With younger stutterers we also have a new speech behavior as our goal and it too is a combination of REEF. The term used with young stutterers is *easy talking.* Concepts involved in each goal are presented below. The controlled fluency or the easy talking deal with the first fear of the stutterer, namely, that he will stutter.

We will *NOT* deal directly with secondary mannerisms. In that they are only associated with stuttering blocks, if blocks do not occur, neither can they. Further, in that the mannerisms play an active role in reducing the fear and anxiety in the stutterer, we would not attempt to remove them unless the stutterer has a new way of speaking which serves the function of reducing the fear and anxiety of speaking.

Rate of speech—(R). Our goal is a slightly slow normal rate of speech, not an exaggeratedly slow speech. The speech rate should sound normal to the listener. I explain this to my clients by drawing an analogy with freeway driving. We set the speed limit at 55 mph and say that the average person talks this fast. However, there are those who talk much faster, say 70 mph, and others who talk much slower at 40 mph. I ask the client to then talk at what he would consider 50 mph. We then shape the speech through verbal and gestural guidance. The normal rate of speech not only gives the stutterer more time for language planning, but also time to make corrections in his speech if a problem arises. With younger clients I explain this by talking about their riding their bikes. If they are riding down a street that has loose gravel on it and a lot of deep holes, they will ride their bikes more slowly so that they do not lose control and fall on the gravel and so they can steer away from the holes. If they ride fast on the street, the would probably skid and fall all on the gravel and would not be able to avoid the holes.

I make the point that the rate of speech is similar to the speed of cars or bikes with both children and adults. Our speed should be determined by how much control we have over our car, our bike, or our mouth. This is determined by the road conditions or the speaking conditions. If a speaking situation has very little stress we might be able to speak at a higher rate, but as the situation becomes more difficult and there is more fear involved, we should slow down to the point where we again have control. The natural tendency of the stutterer is to speak faster in more stressful situations. This would be the same as a driver who increased his speed as the road conditions worsen.

Attending to oral cues—(E). The "E" here stands for "enunciation." This term is used since most clients do not understand when told to attend to proprioceptive and kinesthetic cues. When I attempted to explain this to an older client he said to me, "You mean you want me to enunciate carefully." (A younger client explained it all when he said, "You mean I should talk with my lips.") We will use the term enunciate to mean attending to sensory cues from the mouth or "talk with your lips" with young clients.

Speech is coordinated by interaction between auditory and oral sensory cues. It appears that stutterers attend too much to their auditory cues for speech. When they are deprived of the auditory cues and must rely on oral cues, they no longer stutter. This is the basis of the Edinburgh Masker. When the stutterer starts to speak, the masker is activated and presents a very loud masking tone in both ears of the stutterer, effectively blocking out all other sound. As long as the stutterer can not hear himself speak, he will be fluent. In that he can no longer attend to auditory cues, he shifts to oral cues in order to speak, and the speech is fluent. This same basic principle applies to delayed auditory feedback (DAF). When the auditory cues are delayed, the stutterer must rely more on his oral cues and, again, he is fluent. There are other reasons why the stutterer is fluent on the DAF but we have neither the time nor the space to present them here. Readers who are interested in gaining more insight into the theory and clinical application of the DAF with stutterers are referred to the chapter by Leith and Chmiel (1980). In any event, we have the stutterer use enunciation in order to focus more of his attention on the oral cues, thus decreasing his dependency on auditory monitoring of his speech.

Easy vocal onset—(E). It is not uncommon to see a stutterer attempting to speak while holding his breath. Instead of approximating the vocal folds to the phonatory position, they close them completely, to the breath-holding position. They then increase their subglottal air pressure in an attempt to force vocalization. However, neurologically, they are forcing the folds tighter together since the system is designed to tighten when subglottal air pressure is increased. The harder they push, the tighter the seal becomes. These clients need to be shown how to move the vocal folds from the open position to the phonatory position in a slow and easy fashion. In this way, the folds are prevented from closing beyond the phonatory position. This behavior is commonly taught by having the stutterer vocalize a vowel but to precede it with a "small" (h) sound. He would be asked to say "(h)ay," not the word "hay." By reducing the duration of the (h) sound, the easy vocal onset is established.

Please note that it is not advised to teach the client to introduce speech by taking in a breath and producing the (h) sound to initiate speech. This is just another verbal secondary mannerism, the same thing as getting started on the (uh) sound. The client will end up stuttering on the (h) sound just as he stutters on the (uh) sound.

Smooth flow of speech—(F). The flow of speech is extremely important in stuttering therapy. Most stuttering, about 90%, occurs when the stutterer begins speaking. If the speech is choppy and the stutterer is constantly having to start speech again each time he starts speaking, he has a high probability of stuttering. I explain this by first telling the client that almost all of his stuttering occurs when he starts talking. I then write a sentence, such as, "Mary had a little lamb," and read it as five separate words. When asked how many times I had to start talking, the client will tell me, "Five times." Next, I write the sentence a different way, "Maryhadalittlelamb." When I read it this way, starting only at the beginning, the client will hear me start speech only one time. We then discuss the difference between writing and talking. I explain that we write in words but we talk in "sound trains." We flow all of the words together in a long train of sound, stopping only when we finish a thought, phrase, or idea. By reducing the number of pauses and breaks in the stutterer's speech, we reduce the probability that a stuttering block will occur.

Behaviors to Terminate Blocks

We now turn to those behaviors that we introduce to the older stutterer, not to eliminate the stuttering, but to deal with stuttering blocks if and when they occur. These behaviors address the second fear of the stutterer, that is, how long the block will last once it occurs. There are two basic behavioral strategies the stutterer can turn to to terminate the block.

The glide. The glide is the purposeful, voluntary movement of the articulators from the initial sound of the word to the intermediate vowel. This is a unique form of rate control in that we are slowing down the specific movement of the articulators between the initial sound, or sounds in the case of a blend, to the following vowel. It is a slow and deliberate movement which supersedes the block. The glide appears to influence the language planning of the stutterer during the block, and perhaps the block is the result of disordered language planning. When I introduce the glide I first ask the client to tell me what the sounds are for the letters (b), (d), and (g). Almost without exception, the client will tell me (buh), (duh), and (guh). In other words, they shift from the consonant to the schwa vowel. I then ask them which of the following examples illustrates true stuttering and which is an imitation. Using the word "meet" I say "muh-muh-muh-meet" and "mee-mee-mee-meet." The client usually says that the first example is true stuttering and the second is imitation. The difference is that with actual stuttering, the shift is from the initial sound to the schwa vowel, not the next sound in the word.

I point out that there is no schwa vowel in the word "meet," but the stutterer is trying to say the (m) sound. When asked to say the sound that represents the letter (m), the client will say (muh.) I tell the client that I am going to pretend to take a motion picture of him while he is stuttering on the word "meet." As he is saying, "muh-muh-muh" I take a frame and examine the status of his language planning. The only thing thing I find is the letter "m." The stutterer is telling himself to say the letter (m). And when he does, it comes out (muh). The rest of the word, "eet," is not even in the language plan. The stutterer is totally preoccupied with attempting to say the letter (m), which he does times after time in a repetition without even knowing what the rest of the word is.

With the glide, we are asking the stutterer to think of the rest of the word and to move his articulators into the position of the next vowel. We are forcing him to think of the word, not just the first sound or letter of the word. When he thinks of the rest of the word and slowly moves his articulators to complete the word, he can terminate the block and proceed with the word. With younger stutterers I have used the analogy of sliding into second base in a baseball game. I tell them to "slide" into the rest of the word. This seems to get the concept across.

Words that begin with a vowel present another problem. But now we use easy onset with the glide; the gradual introduction of vocalization and the slow shift to the rest of the word. You might even look at easy onset as a form of the glide which the client uses when he is faced with a block on a vowel rather than a consonant.

Stop/correct. This technique has a built in danger of becoming a "retrial" where the stutterer simply stops, backs up a few words, and tries to say the stuttered word again. I insist that the stutterer change his speech behavior when he uses this technique, that is, when he starts speaking again he must use his REEF. The block occurred because he was not using his new speech behavior. When he starts again, using his REEF, the probability of the block occurring is greatly reduced. Great care must be taken to ensure that the stutterer does not just repeat the initial word or phrase, using the old speech behavior and performing a retrial. If done properly, this is a good form of cancellation, cancelling the practice of the incorrect speech behavior with a practice of the correct speech behavior.

The stutterer can also use the glide with his stop/correct technique. For example, the stutterer has said, "My name is FFFF" and then stopped. He then repeats the phrase using his REEF and, when he says his name "Fred," he uses the glide. In this use of the glide, the stutterer is preventing the stuttering from occurring. In that he just stuttered on his name and his fear of the word is heightened, he applies the glide as another precaution against the stuttering reoccurring. Thus, the glide can be used either to terminate a block that has occurred or, by gliding on a feared word, to prevent the stuttering from occurring.

Chapter 5

Cognitive Aspects of Stuttering

THE STUTTERER'S COGNITIVE SET

Now that we have examined the behavioral aspects of stuttering, let us consider the effects that these behaviors have on the individual who stutters. When we discuss the stutterer's cognitive set, we are referring to how the stutterer views himself, how he views his stuttering, his attitudes, his beliefs, his fears, anxiety, and other such cognitive factors. This is the "psyche" of the stutterer. All of these "sets" are learned. The stutterer was not born with these "sets," they were learned as he experienced the problems his stuttering was creating in his life.

At the root of this process is the stuttering. It is the source of the fear, the anxiety, the shame, the anger, the frustration. It influences every aspect of the stutterer's thinking. All aspects of the stutterer's life are involved in stuttering, either directly or indirectly. The extent of the stutterer's emotional involvement in his stuttering is difficult to comprehend, even for the speech clinician, but we must attempt to understand it if we are to work clinically with stutterers.

In our view of stuttering, both the stuttering behaviors themselves and the cognitive set of the stutterer are involved. In our therapy, we also view both the stuttering behaviors and the stutterer's cognitive set of learned behaviors. Therefore, we will deal with both in our therapy, working with the *stuttering* and the *stutterer.* This is counter to most pure behavioral approaches to stuttering where the theory is that once the stuttering is "eliminated," the negative cognitive set of the stutterer will correct itself. The cognitive set is viewed as a "symptom" of stuttering and once the stuttering is "removed," the symptom will disappear. One problem with this line of reasoning is that the stuttering can never be totally eliminated or removed. This would constitute a "cure" and there is no known cure for stuttering. Another problem with this reasoning is illustrated in the following analogy.

Let us consider an extremely homely child. Her years in school were miserable with being teased and shunned. This same theme continued through college and then, at the age of 23, she had plastic surgery. The surgery resulted in an average-looking woman, neither homely nor beautiful. No one approached her and rewarded her by telling her how beautiful she was. She was simply accepted as an average-looking woman. But, her self-concept, after all of the years of rejection, remained that of being homely. She even saw herself that way in a mirror. Her cognitive set did not change since there were no rewards to change it. Change might occur over a long period of time but this would also be partially dependent on her receiving compliments on her appearance from her social contacts.

A parallel can be drawn here with the stutterer who has achieved normal-sounding speech. He will still have a poor self-concept. He does not receive rewards for his speech except from his closest friends, and even they stop doing this after a short period of time. To the average listener he has normal-sounding speech but not outstanding or deserving of a reward. Recognizing that we are unable to totally eliminate stuttering and that the stutterer's cognitive set may not change even with improved speech, we deal with the cognitive set directly.

Development of the Cognitive Set: Influence of the Stuttering

Listener's reactions. The first reactions to the stuttering that the child is exposed to are, most likely, those of the parents and siblings. How do most parents react to stuttering? They can either reward it or penalize it and, with very few exceptions, they often penalize it one way or another. Regardless of the often-heard advice to ignore the stuttering, there is no such thing. It is impossible to ignore. The parents will have some reaction to the stuttering, no matter how subtle. Many parents feel that, if they stand still and do not say anything about the stuttering, they are not reacting, even though they may have a look of horror on their faces. Children learn to read their parent's body language at a very early age. The child may not know that the parents are reacting to his speech, but he will know that something is wrong. And then there are those parents who directly penalize the stuttering through either verbal or physical abuse. The reasons for parental response are discussed later in this chapter.

Siblings also become involved in creating the cognitive set in the stutterer. If a sibling gets into an argument with the child who stutters, there is nothing quite as convenient to pick on as the stuttering. He can be called names, his speech can be imitated, he can be teased—and the stutterer has no verbal defenses.

Peers are also a factor in the development of the cognitive set. They are, in a special way, different from siblings and parents and often more influential. Peers have the same means of upsetting the stutterer as do the siblings: calling him names, imitating his speech, and teasing him. Although peer pressure is present in every phase of the stutterer's life, it is especially important as the stutterer goes through adolescence.

When we talk about "other listeners" we mean those people the stutterer must talk to in order to survive in society. These people are teachers, counselors, clerks in stores, bus drivers, telephone operators, and others the stutterer might talk to. Although these people are not in constant contact with the stutterer, they do have an impact on the development of the stutterer's cognitive set through their reactions to the stuttering. Often their reactions may be totally neutral but the stutterer, looking for a negative reaction, will "see" one even though it did not exist. This is an extremely important point. If the stutterer feels someone is reacting negatively to him and his speech, then it is true in his mind and must be dealt with as a "fact." There is a bit of "paranoia" in the stutterer and the speech clinician must recognize its existence and deal with it clinically.

Failure in self-improvement of speech. With all stutterers we see, they will have attempted to modify their speech. This is the origin of secondary mannerisms. With each mannerism that the stutterer adopts, he feels that he has at last cured himself of his stuttering. Then the effectiveness of the mannerism decreases and the stuttering returns. He then adopts another mannerism and the process is repeated time after time as the stuttering develops. All of this failure creates a defeatist attitude. The stutterer begins to believe that he is a victim, with no way to escape from the stuttering. This belief has a profound effect on the stutterer's cognitive set about his speech, about himself, and about any therapy he receives.

As the stutterer matures, the problem of self-concept and self-confidence become more pronounced. He becomes increasingly aware of the social and economic implications of his stuttering. He has also had additional time to develop more secondary mannerisms, more fears, and more failures in therapy. He develops a negative attitude toward himself and his ability to deal with the stuttering and becomes extremely critical of himself and the ways he deals with and reacts to his speech.

Failure in therapy. To confound the picture even more, most of the clients we see have been through therapy before and failed. Had they not failed, they would not be back in therapy. Here is another defeat, another failure. This presents us with a serious problem since the stutterer has previously worked with a speech clinician and she did not resolve the stuttering. Not only are we faced with his feelings of defeat and failure, he is also suspicious of us and our therapy. He has been through it before, perhaps many times and over a long period of time, and the therapy has failed. His experiences in therapy have not provided him with what he is seeking, that is, to be cured. He entered into therapy believing that he would leave therapy without a stuttering problem. But he is back in therapy again since the therapy did not eliminate the problem. There is a gap between what the stutterer expects from therapy and what he receives. This is referred to as "cognitive dissonance."

These clinical "failures" tend to support the stutterer's belief that he is a "victim" of stuttering and that there is nothing that can be done about it. He is helpless. And yet, he still seeks help. This is the intellectual side of the stutterer. He knows that he needs assistance so he goes seeking it. But the emotional side of the stutterer "knows" that the therapy will not help since there is nothing that can be done; it is a helpless situation. There is an obvious conflict between the intellectual and the emotional sides of the stutterer. This presents problems for both the stutterer and the clinician.

Grieving over loss. In attempting to understand and work with the cognitive set of the stutterer, I turned to the five stages of grief associated with loss (Kubler-Ross, 1969; Westburg, 1962). What has the stutterer lost? He has lost the ability to speak like other people.

The stages of grief are denial, anger, bargaining, depression, and acceptance. When we apply these stages to the stutterer we, and perhaps the stutterer, can gain some insight into why he thinks as he does. The stage of *denial* means that while some stutterers actually deny that they are stutterers, others deny that their stuttering is a problem or that it will be with them the rest of their lives. To better understand how a stutterer could deny his problem, recognize that, if you carefully analyze the speech of any stutterer, you will find that most of the speech is fluent. It would be rare to find a stutterer who stuttered on more than 50% of the words spoken. In many instances, even with the most severe stutterers, there are situations where the speech is totally fluent such as when singing, talking to younger persons or talking to animals. It is not too difficult to imagine the stutterer denying he is actually a stutterer, or that it is a problem, or that it will be one for the rest of his life.

The second stage is *anger* and most stutterers are angry. They are angry because they have lost the ability to speak fluently. They ask, "Why me?" They are looking for someone to blame for their affliction. They are angry with themselves for not having the courage to confront their stuttering and for allowing the stuttering to dominate their lives. They are angry because they cannot say what they want to say. There is also a lot of anger directed to listeners who, in their mind, respond negatively to them when they stutter by means such as saying the word for them or looking away.

In the third stage, *bargaining,* the stutterer bargains in several ways. Some pray that the stuttering will be taken away in exchange for a commitment on their part to do something. One client, a minister, prayed that if his stuttering was cured he would go into the ministry. He summarized the results of the bargain when he said that both he and God lost since he still stutters and God has a stuttering minister. The stutterer also bargains with the clinician. His bargain is that if he faithfully attends all of the therapy sessions, the clinician will assume the responsibility for "curing" him of his stuttering.

The fourth stage is *depression.* The stutterer, after repeated attempts to free himself of the stuttering, finds that he cannot get rid of it and becomes depressed. This is a common emotion with all stutterers, especially those who have been through several therapy programs and who still stutter.

The final stage is *acceptance.* Here, the stutterer finally accepts the fact that he is and will always be a stutterer. He recognizes that there is no known cure for stuttering. He also discovers that therapy can help him by reducing the severity of the stuttering to the point where it is no longer a major negative influence in his life. He then applies all of the energy he wasted worrying about it to actively working on his speech in therapy.

Unfortunately, the stutterer does not progress through these stages and then settle in acceptance. He constantly goes back and forth through the stages but, as therapy progresses, he spends less and less time in the stages of denial, anger, bargaining, and depression. As the stutterer is in the various stages, there will be differing degrees of clinical resistance.

Influence of the Stutterer's Culture

We are concerned here with the demands made of the stutterer by his cultural group, that is, what is expected of him in terms of cultural behaviors and beliefs. Various cultural groups have a lifestyle based on their cultural heritage and this may be quite distinct from what might be called "general American" culture. However, do not overgeneralize with cultural groups. You must consider each individual separately and not judge the person by your preconceived ideas of his general cultural group. Other factors you must consider are the degree of assimilation into the general American culture, the socioeconomic level, the educational level, the influence of religion, and so forth. Consider, for example, the pressure exerted on the stutterer in those cultures which emphasize verbal skills. Consider the effect on the female stutterer in those cultures where the female with any sort of "defect" is scorned. Consider eye contact, a major concern of many stuttering therapies. There are several cultures which view eye contact as an act of hostility, a behavior not to be performed in normal social interactions.

We cannot discuss all of the numerous cultures and their differences but I would strongly recommend that you become somewhat familiar with the cultural background of your clients. I would further recommend that you read the article on cultural influences in stuttering by Leith and Mims (1975) and the chapter on this subject by Leith (in preparation).

Maintenance of the Cognitive Set

Continued failure. The experiences the stutterer has with his attempts to change his speech, either through self-modification (usually secondary mannerisms) or through therapy, continue to be negative. He attempts to deal with his speech but continues to fail, thus strengthening his belief that he is a victim of the stuttering. This belief becomes stronger over time since the failures continue.

Increased fear and anxiety. The more helpless the stutterer feels, the more fear and anxiety he develops about talking situations. Because he has failed to modify the stuttering, he becomes anxious about talking situations, fearing that the stuttering will occur. Different situations take on differing amounts of fear and the more fear there is in a situation, the more he stutters. The fear of specific talking situations also generalizes to other similar situations. The stutterer may develop great difficulty in talking to a clerk in a particular store. This would then generalize to fear of talking to clerks in any store.

Listener reactions. Having developed a bit of "paranoia" about the reactions of listeners to his stuttering, the stutterer continues to see these reactions when he stutters. Thus, his belief that listeners are responding negatively to him is strengthened with each speaking experience where he stutters.

Helplessness. The longer the stutterer experiences failure in his attempts to modify his speech, the more helpless he feels. Nothing that he or a speech clinician can do will remove the stuttering. The feeling of being a victim is strengthened over time.

Lack of emotional growth. It would appear that the negative emotional response to the stuttering reaches its peak during the sensitive adolescent years. However, even though the stutterer may mature physically, there seems to be no emotional growth, that is, the stutterer continues to react to his stuttering as he did during his teenage years. He does not develop an adult view of the stuttering, developing the courage to face the stuttering and deal with it on a less emotional level.

Effects of Cognitive Set on Therapy

Although the stutterer may seek out therapy, the motivation is tempered by the memories of previous failures. The stutterer may not be willing to take the risk necessary for successful therapy since he has a fear of failing again. He approaches therapy with caution and is looking for any failure that might occur. The clinician must work against this "set." One of the most common signs of this fear of failure is the lack of true commitment by the stutterer to the therapy. He will be resistant to various therapy strategies and will not carry out work assignments outside the clinical environment. *Basically, the stutterer does not trust himself or the therapy.* He has failed too many times in the past to accept any therapy at face value. Our main clinical tasks are to cultivate the existing motivation, to maintain it during therapy, and to change the cognitive set.

The problems discussed above are even more serious when we consider the stutterer who is sent for therapy by his parents, a teacher, or some other person. This stutterer enters therapy not only with no motivation but also with all of the negative emotions of the stutterers who seek therapy. Our problems are now even greater since we must not only create motivation in this client, but we must also maintain it. Our only tools to create motivation with this type of client are the rewards and penalties we administer in our therapy as set forth in the CIM in chapter 2.

With both types of clients we must include, as part of our therapy, the modification of the cognitive set. As the cognitive set is changed to a more positive orientation, there will be a reflected increase in motivation to work on the stuttering and a commitment to therapy.

Evaluation of Cognitive Set

There are no formal scales or procedures for evaluating the stutterer's cognitive set. There are some scales that address the amount of fear the stutterer associates with various speaking situations but this is only a small part of the total picture of the stutterer's cognitive set. There are several informal scales that address the stutterer's set toward his stuttering, but this information cannot be achieved in one or two clinical sessions. It surfaces slowly over time in therapy. The clinician must ask very specific questions and listen carefully to the stutterer's response. Even then the clinician must sift through the stutterer's responses and determine their credibility. For example, if the clinician asks the stutterer if his stuttering bothers him and his response is, "No, it never bothers me," the clinician should not accept this statement at face value. The stutterer might find it demeaning to admit that his stuttering bothers him. This could well be a cultural factor. The clinician should recognize that many stutterers need to protect their self-concept by denying that the stuttering bothers them or that they are afraid of it. Further, if the stuttering did not "bother" the stutterer, he would not have developed any secondary mannerisms or, for that matter, would not even be coming for therapy.

One might expect that there would be a direct relationship between the severity of the stuttering and the severity of the stutterer's emotional reaction to it. I have not found this to be true. I have worked with some severe stutterers who had a "mild" emotional reaction to it. I have also worked with some mild stutterers who had a "severe" emotional reaction to the stuttering. The emotional reaction seems to be coming from two different sources. Some stutterers, usually the more severe stutterers, fear their stuttering since they might not be able to say what they want to say while others, the more mild stutterers who have little difficulty saying what they want to say, fear that someone will find out that they are a stutterer.

The severity of the stuttering and the emotional response of the client to his stuttering will have a direct bearing on the efficiency and effectiveness of our therapy. However, there is no way to predict the outcome of therapy since we do not know the relationship between these factors and since there are still other factors involved. You are best advised to be aware that the severity of stuttering and emotional reactions to it may influence your therapy and deal with these factors if and when they pose problems in therapy. You can deal with this best by approaching the client's cognitive set through the techniques which follow.

Techniques to Change Cognitive Set

There are a number of ways we can approach the problem of changing the cognitive set of the stutterer. The techniques can be used individually or in any combination and all are applied through the CIM.

Information about stuttering. Most stutterers do not have any insight into their problem. They do not understand what is happening to them, why it is happening, or why they feel as they do. The more information the client has about stuttering and the better he understands it, the less fear and anxiety he associates with it. The client should be told that stuttering is learned—not the actual repetitions and prolongations, but the fear of talking. With increased fear and tension, the greater the likelihood is that stuttering will occur. Secondary mannerisms should be explained in terms of things that he does to avoid stuttering, and that after a short period of time they no longer prevent the stuttering from occurring. However, they continue to exist, making the stuttering blocks more complex and more socially unacceptable. An analogy I have used concerns a two-layer cake. The first layer is "repetitions" and the second layer is "prolongations." When the stutterer adopts the first mannerism it becomes the first layer of frosting on the cake. When this mannerism is no longer effective, another mannerism is adopted and this becomes the second layer of frosting. This process continues as more and more layers of frosting are put on the cake. The number of layers of frosting are dependent on the individual stutterer.

The client should also understand where the block occurs in his speech. Most stutterers feel that they stutter on specific sounds. It is very important that they understand that they stutter on the movements *between* sounds, not on the sounds themselves. I demonstrate this with the following illustration:

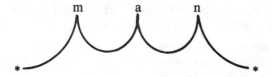

I then explain that when I say the word I start with my mouth in a neutral position (*), move the articulators into the (m) sound, move them into the (a) sound, move into the (n) sound, and then move back in the neutral position (*). Once this is understood I then stutter on the word, "muh-muh-muh-man," and ask the client where the block occurred. The client will usually say that I stuttered on the (m) sound. I point out that I said the (m) sound four times but I did not move my mouth into the (a) sound. Instead of the (a) sound, I said the (uh) sound, the schwa vowel which does not even exist in the word. My next example of stuttering is "uh-uh-uh-man," I explain that with this type of block I did not move my mouth out of the neutral position (the schwa vowel) into the (m) sound. My last example is "mmmmmmmmmman." Again, I did not move out of the (m) sound into the (a) sound. This concept of where the block occurs in words is very important in that part of our therapy will be based on teaching the client to voluntarily move his articulators from one position to another to avoid or terminate stuttering blocks.

While discussing the articulatory positioning of the mouth, it is very common for the stutterer to be attempting to say a sound but not to have his mouth in the position to say the sound. He may be attempting to say the (m) sound but he is attempting to produce it with his mouth wide open. I tell the stutterer that if he must stutter, to at least stutter on the right sound and that if the mouth is in the correct position, chances are that the block will not occur.

Finally, I point out to the stutterer that, even with his most feared words, he does not stutter on them 100% of the time. There is no sound or word that he stutters on consistently. He can always say the sound or word in some context. I also point out that no matter how severe the stutterer is, a good share of his speech is fluent. It is rare to find a stutterer so severe that he stutters on more than 50% of his words. This means he is fluent 50% of the time when he is speaking.

With clients who have some reading skills, I have them read a book dealing with the emotional acceptance of stuttering, *What Can I Do About the Part of Me I Don't Like?* by David R. Belgum (1974). Dr. Belgum is both a minister and a stutterer and presents the reader with the challenges he faced as he dealt with accepting his own stuttering. My clients have enjoyed the book and have gained a lot of insight into how they are dealing with their own stuttering.

Listener reactions to stuttering. Stutterers have two basic fears, fear that they will stutter and, when they are actually in a stuttering block, how long the block will last. The most obvious question is, what is the stutterer afraid of? When we get to the core, we will find that the stutterer fears his listener's reaction to his stuttering. He feels that, when he stutters, his listener thinks he is "stupid," "weird," "strange," "retarded," or something equally negative. The stutterer is watching for these negative reactions in his listeners, and he will see them, even if they truly do not exist. For example, if the stutterer is talking to someone and they happen to look away for a second, the stutterer will interpret this as the listener's negative reaction to his stuttering. He would not consider that the breaking of eye contact by the listener might be due to some other, unrelated reason.

I have found that the best way to approach this is to first point out that the average listener knows nothing about stuttering and does not know how to react when the stuttering occurs. If a listener does indeed look away during a block, he might be trying, in his own way, to relieve the pressure on the stutterer. It is not socially acceptable behavior to stare **at** something unusual. If someone has a birthmark on their face, one does not sit and stare at it. When a stutterer has a block, the same social standard is applied; one does not stare at it. The stutterer should at least recognize that the listener's intentions were good.

How does the listener decide how to react to stuttering? The stutterer tells him. When the stutterer is embarrassed by a stuttering block and manifests it overtly, the listener is uneasy and embarrassed since he is involved in the stutterer's embarrassment. The stutterer's struggle behavior signals his attitude about his stuttering. His listener reads this and responds accordingly. How do listeners react when they are uneasy or embarrassed? Some may look away, others may laugh. Each listener handles his uneasiness or embarrassment individually. If the stutterer is truly not embarrassed with his stuttering, the listener will not be either.

The stutterer is upset with many of his listeners since they are not understanding or patient with him. And yet he does not extend the same courtesy to his listeners. He is not understanding of their plight nor patient with their attempts to respond appropriately to the stuttering. With many stutterers, their goal is to "fool" everyone into believing that the stuttering does not bother them. They put on a mask to cover up their true feelings about their stuttering. When they are successful with the charade and the listener, believing what is seen and heard, responds accordingly, they become angry with the listener for being insensitive. Who is creating all of the problems in these interpersonal relationships? In most instances it is the stutterer himself. If the stutterer can recognize his role in this, his attitude toward his listeners will be modified and this will lessen the fear and anxiety associated with talking situations.

Counseling. We have already discussed the influence of the five stages of grief on the stutterer. Now we should discuss them with him. We can discuss his denial of the problem, allow him to express his anger about being a stutterer, deal with his bargaining, and allow him to express his depression. Through the expression of this "negative emotion," he may resolve some of his problems. We can nod, we can agree, we can present information that is counter to some of his feelings, we can be quiet and allow him to vent the feelings. Through this counseling and success in therapy, we can shift his cognitive set to the last stage, that of acceptance, thus, shift all of the energy he spent worrying about his stuttering to working on controlling it.

The relationship between you and the client during counseling is based on the CIM model. However, in this application, you are going to have the client do most of the talking. Your stimulus will usually be in the form of a question or a request for the client to expand on or further clarify something he has said. If you want to disagree with something he has said in order for him to see another viewpoint, you can also provide information or opinions. If you review the CIM model you will see how it provides you with a guide for counseling your client.

Inventory of assets. Since the stutterer has a negative outlook on life in general, he usually focuses on what he sees as his liabilities. The stutterer should be asked to make up a list of his assets, those things about him that are positive. This is difficult since the stutterer has spent so much time dwelling on the liabilities, real and imagined, that he has ignored the positive aspects of himself and his personality. I have my stutterers make out a list of assets and then we discuss them. I add to the list if I see other assets and then expand on each asset in the discussion. I provide support for the assets by praising (rewarding) these aspects of the stutterer.

Group sharing. Most stutterers have not had the opportunity to share their "sets" with other stutterers. They feel that they are alone in their fears, their avoidances, their anxiety. If several stutterers are put together in a group setting there is the opportunity for them to share their feelings, attitudes, beliefs, and so forth. They are usually surprised to find that there are other people who feel exactly as they do. They then no longer feel that they have strange or abnormal "sets." They learn that this is part of being a stutterer. As the group begins to share feelings, each stutterer will gain some insight into why he feels as he does. Each stutterer will have a somewhat different view of the factors influencing his cognitive set and, when offered several views of the same factor, the stutterer's cognitive set cannot help but be influenced. Through group sharing, changes in the clients' cognitive sets will occur. This cannot be done in a group where there is only one stutterer. Clients with other types of communication disorders will not understand the stutterer's feelings.

Record keeping. Because the stutterer is preoccupied with his speech failures, we must counterbalance this by focusing him on his successes with speech. I start this early in therapy by keeping a record of better speech in the clinic room. As the client begins to use his new speech behavior, I reward his new speech whenever it occurs. This is part of shaping, the gradual changing of the speech to the new speech behavior. I make a note of the amount of reward the client has received and then discuss this with him at the end of each session, showing him clearly that he is succeeding in making his speech more fluent. I stress his success in order to change the "set" of failure and helplessness.

When I feel the new speech behavior is stable enough to test in controlled situations outside the clinic room, I introduce the client to the "log book." This is a record of the practice the client does as he takes his new speech behavior out of the clinical environment. I discuss the log book with the client and give him a set of written instructions on the use of the log book. These instructions will be found in Appendix A. The instructions in the appendix may have to be simplified for younger stutterers. We use a different record keeping system for the very young stutterer. This is discussed later in the chapter.

Before the stutterer begins to use the log book, we must establish a few ground rules. First, I establish a psychological stress hierarchy of speaking situations. I ask the client what his easiest talking situation is. If this is talking at home, I label this a "1" situation. I then ask what the most difficult situation is. When the client identifies this, such as reciting in class, I label this is a "5" situation. We then establish "2," "3," and "4' situations. The client can then relate to me how much stress he is under in any situation by simply identifying it as a 3 or a 5.

We must determine a method of grading the speech. With the new speech behavior, the stutterer will still have some stuttering dysfluencies in his speech but they will not be what would be considered traditional blocks. Rather, the stutterer will have what we refer to as a "sticky." The sticky is an effortless, short prolongation which terminates with a smooth glide into the rest of the word. It is as if the speech system "sticks" or "hangs up" for an instant. If the stutterer is not using his new speech behavior, he will have more traditional blocks.

The grading system is based on the "normality" of speech. If the speech flows well, has a normal rate, and there is only an occasional very short sticky (about one-half second), the speech grade would be an "A." A listener would not be aware that there was anything "different" about the speech. Speech at the "B" level would not flow quite as smooth and the rate might be slightly too fast. The stickies would be a bit longer and would occur more often but still not interfere with the speech. The listener would also consider this normal speech. When the flow of speech is slightly choppy, the rate noticeably too fast, and the stickies long enough that they are interfering slightly with the speech, the speech is graded "C." The listener would consider the talker to be dysfluent but not a stutterer since there is not struggle behavior, no pushing to get the word out. The dysfluency is still a sticky, not a "raw" block. When the stutterer is not using his new speech behavior, he will have stuttering blocks rather than stickies. The struggle behavior is obvious. But, if the stutterer is able to terminate his blocks by gliding into the rest of the word, the grade for the speech is a "D" since he does have some control over the speech. This listener would now label the client a stutterer. The "E" grade is used when the client uses no controls with his speech. The stuttering blocks run their course as the stutterer struggles to get the word out. Thus, the grading system differentiates between *normal* (grades of A and B), *dysfluent* speech (grade of C), and *stuttering* speech (grades D and E). I check my clients' grading system by having them grade their speech in the clinic room and compare their grades with mine. If our grades differ too much, we discuss the system and try again. I check the grading system about once every 2 weeks to make sure the client is still using the same criteria for his speech grades.

Once these criteria are established, the client is required to perform and record in the log book one or two practice speaking situations per day. It is suggested that he limit his practice to lower stress situations (1, 2, or 3 situations). Each practice is limited to approximately 10 seconds because the stutterer must memorize what he is going to say in the situation and this is about as much as a person can memorize quickly. By doing this, the client does not have to think of WHAT he is going to say, he can concentrate on HOW he is saying it. A speech practice is differentiated from a speech "game." Speech games last longer and are spontaneous rather than preplanned. This means that the client is attending more to WHAT he is saying than on HOW he is saying it. We do not want any speech games in the log book early in therapy, only practices. We include games only after the client is consistently getting grades of "A" in 1 and 2 situations. When games are used, they tell us how well the client can use the new speech behavior over an extended period of time when he is not focusing on it.

The client is to practice one aspect of his new speech behavior in each situation and record the results. He first identifies the situation so that he can remember it later, then rates the stress of the situation as he enters it. This is done before he actually speaks in the situation. After he has completed the talking situation he finishes the log book by rating the stress when he was finished, grading his speech, and noting which aspect of the speech behavior he was concentrating on. The log book is then brought to therapy and reviewed by the clinician. You may have to spend a session or two straightening out errors in recording the practices such as not including games, recording the correct stress level, and other entries. Once the client has learned how to record his practices, a typical log book might appear as follows:

Monday

1. Asked Mary question
2. 2

1. Bought a coke
2. 3

3. 2   3. 2
4. B−   4. B
5. Rate   5. Enunciation

In both practice situations the client has been able to improve his speech from an E, his old speech, to a B− and a B. This is quite an improvement since he was not perceived as a "stutterer" in either situation. Further, he anticipated a 3 stress level when he ordered a coke but, since his speech was under such good control, the situational stress reduced to a 2. These successes should be pointed out to him and he should be rewarded for the good work he did on his speech.

As the data in the log book are collected over time, you will be able to see improvement not only from the standpoint of better speech grades but the stress associated with various speaking situations will also be reduced. Analysis of the log book should show the speech grades improving, first in the less stressful situations and then in the more difficult ones. You should also see, over time, reduction in stress during situations, as shown in the situation above where the client bought a coke. As confidence builds you will also see a reduction in anticipated stress, as when the client above orders another coke and his anticipated stress, item #2, is recorded as a 2 rather than a 3. When the anticipated stress is reduced from its original level it means that some significant changes are occurring in the client's cognitive set. Finally, a review of the speech grades will indicate how many of his practices resulted in normal-sounding speech. If the log book is introduced at the proper time in therapy, during the generalization phase, most of the situational speech should be normal-sounding and show grades not less than a C. You should do this analysis carefully and completely with the client at least once every 2 weeks. Emphasize the positive changes that are occurring and reward the client for his efforts and his successes. This is the way we use the log book to change the cognitive set and maintain motivation.

When the client is able to consistently get grades of C or better in all situations, we now have the client enter some speech games into the log book, listing the same data plus making a note of how long the game lasted. The game data are very important in the modification of the stutterer's cognitive set since we are now showing him that he can use the new speech behavior over a period of time in spontaneous talking situations.

The size of the log book is an important factor. It should be small enough to be carried in a pocket since the client is expected to carry it with him at all times so he can write down his practices immediately rather than wait and depend on how well he remembers the practice. The log book plays many roles as we generalize the new speech behavior. Since the client carries it with him at all times, it reminds him to try to use his new speech behavior, and the glide and stop/correct techniques. Because we are rewarding the reports of practices in the log book, it becomes an S+, prompting the new speech behaviors to occur. If we penalize the client when his log book assignments are not completed, the log book also becomes an S−, cuing the client to do his assignments in order to avoid the penalty.

With the preschool and the very early elementary client, I also keep a record of successes, much as I do with the older client. The log book is not applicable here because of the cognitive level of the clients, a more subtle clinical approach to the stuttering, and the lack of writing skills.

When the parents are working with me, I have them keep a record book, a recording of how many rewards the client receives for using his new speech behavior, easy talking, and in what talking situations the easy talking is occurring. Although not as thorough or as "objective" as the log book, it can be used in the same way, to point out to the young stutterer that he is able to speak more fluently. Again, we use the record book to change the stutterer's cognitive set, to show him that he can speak without stuttering. This is accomplished by both the parents' and our reviewing the record book with the client.

Without parental involvement in the therapy program, we are limited to a record book that we keep during therapy. This is a poor substitute for a record book kept by parents but it is the best we can do. Other people in the client's life, such as a teacher, may be able to assist in keeping records and this will be discussed in the therapy section dealing with the young child.

With early elementary clients I have them keep a record book, using symbols to indicate where they practiced their easy talking and how successful it was. Since we are dealing with clients with limited writing skills, I have the clients use symbols to indicate where they practiced and how well they did. One client used stick figures to remember who he talked to (his mother had long hair, his father had a beard, his teacher had glasses) and happy, neutral, and sad faces to remind him of how well he was able to use his easy talking. He worked out a rather elaborate system of symbols so that he could report his practices to me and to his parents. This type of record book must be worked out for each client according to his skills and cognitive ability.

Professional referrals. In some instances you will find a client whose cognitive set is so negative that therapy on a continuing basis is impossible. You have two choices. You can either terminate the stuttering therapy and make a referral for counseling or you can continue your therapy while the client is also receiving counseling. In either event, you must coordinate your activities with the counselor so that you can take appropriate action if there is a significant change in the client's cognitive set.

THE PARENTS' COGNITIVE SET

The aspect of the parents' cognitive set which concerns us most is their attitude toward their child's stuttering. They will have formed some idea of why their child stutters and if they played a part in it. This will form the basis of how they respond to the child when he stutters. If the parents feel that it is just that the child is being "stubborn," and talking that way to annoy them, their responses to the stuttering will be quite negative, usually one of frustration and anger. If, on the other hand, they believe that their child stutters because of something that they have done, they react in a different way, showing their anxiety and guilt. It is also possible that some parents may have a neutral and objective cognitive set toward their child's stuttering. However, most parents will be emotionally involved in the problem. Since the parents are involved, either directly or indirectly, in our therapy their cognitive sets have a direct bearing on the efficiency and effectiveness of our treatment program.

Development of the Cognitive Set

The attitudes, beliefs, and emotions of the parents are shaped by the guilt most parents feel when they discover their child has some sort of defect or problem. The parents feel that, in some way, they caused the problem. In the case of stuttering, the parents do play a part in creating stuttering but, since we do not know the cause of stuttering, we cannot determine how significant their role was. Further, we do not know all of the other factors that play a part in bringing about stuttering in children. Still, most parents have some guilt about their possible role in their child's stuttering.

In addition to the guilt, most parents are also angry and frustrated. Their anger is directed both toward the fact that it is their child who stutters but also, in many cases, toward the child himself. The child is a source of great frustration since the parents do not know what to do or how to respond when he stutters. In some instances, the parents are very embarrassed about their child's stuttering, feeling perhaps that it is a reflection of their parenting. Suffice it to say that most parents develop some degree of a negative set regarding their child and his stuttering.

When we apply the five stages of grief to the parents, we can also gain some insight into why the parents develop a negative cognitive set. They too have lost something: a "normal" child. They deny that their child has a serious speech problem. They may, indeed, believe that the child is stuttering on purpose and this belief makes them angry with the child. At the same time they are angry that their child can not speak like other children. They are angry that it is their child who is so afflicted. And, yes, they also bargain either through prayer or with the district and/or the clinician. They are deeply involved in the failure of the child to "outgrow" the problem or be "cured" in therapy. They are depressed with the entire situation. It is extremely difficult for them to accept their child's stuttering.

Maintenance of the Cognitive Set

The negative cognitive set is maintained, or even magnified, over the years. The primary source of this is the developmental nature of the stuttering itself. The stuttering gets more severe over time as the stutterer develops more secondary mannerisms, more fears, and so on. So, in the eyes of the parents, and as a matter of fact, the stuttering continues to become more severe as time passes.

Another factor that maintains the parents' negative cognitive set is their continuing failure to find a "cure" for their child's stuttering. The family physician tells them one with thing to do while friends tell them another. None of the advice resolves the stuttering problem. If the child has also received stuttering therapy, again, there was no "cure" for the stuttering. The parents feel helpless, not knowing where to turn or what to do. This is a major source of frustration, anger, and guilt.

Effects of Cognitive Set on Therapy

The influence of parental cognitive set on therapy is related to the age of the stutterer. With older stutterers, the set of the parents may have little or no influence. However, with younger stutterers the parental set becomes increasingly important. The parental set will determine if a home program will be established and if the child will receive support from the parents as he works on his stuttering.

We deal with three possible parental sets with regard to therapy. If the parental set is positive and they are cooperative and work with us, our clinical job is much easier. However, if the parents' set is neutral and they are uncooperative, we face many clinical problems. These parents may approve of their child receiving therapy, but they will not cooperate in terms of working with the child at home since they do not feel it is really a problem. They are neither working with us or against us. The most disruptive effect of the parental set is where the parents penalize the child for stuttering. The penalty may result from the parent's frustration, which is expressed in anger or, perhaps, they penalize the child because they feel he is stuttering on purpose. In either situation, our therapy will suffer directly since, because of their attitudes, these parents are working against our attempt to reverse the child's negative set.

Techniques to Change the Cognitive Set

If the cognitive set of the parents is creating clinical problems for us, we must try to change it. We will use many of the same techniques we use to change the stutterer's cognitive set. The main problem in changing the set of parents is the limited access the school clinician has to the client's parents. Some parents will come in for a conference and, in this instance, we want to provide them with as much information about stuttering as possible, including giving them appropriate ways to react when their child stutters. There are also books and pamphlets that the parents can read. Several of these are listed in the References and Recommended Readings. (These are important resources you can also use with parents who cannot or will not come in for a conference.) During the conference, it is important to deal with the cause of stuttering. Most parents, whether they verbalize it or not, have some guilt feelings about their "causing" their child to stutter. I counsel parents by explaining that we really do not know what causes stuttering. There are many factors which must be present in order for a child to begin to stutter and we are not sure of what all of the factors are. I then tell the parents that if, when their child was born, they had decided to make him stutter, they could not have done it. I feel it is very important to deal with the parents' guilt and relieve as much of it as possible and a discussion of stuttering, its origins and implications, should help change the set of parents who are willing to come in for a conference. For these parents who are unable or unwilling to come in for a conference, information about stuttering can be sent to them. A "letter" to such parents is found in Appendix B. This letter can be modified according to your unique clinical needs.

If we have access to the parents we should also attempt to deal with the stages of grief mentioned in the development of the cognitive set. As with the stutterer, we can allow the parents to express their feelings and their frustrations about the stuttering. As we provide the parents with information about stuttering, this may help change their sets in some of the stages. We can also provide some support for their concerns for their child. Our interactions with the parents at this level can only yield a positive result. Our best tactic may be to just let the parents talk out their feelings and concerns.

—NOTES—

We face a different problem with those parents who cannot come in to discuss their child's problem. We can use the telephone as a substitute for an in-person conference. This will be a relatively good substitute for the direct conference. You can present the information about stuttering and how to react to it to the parents and discuss it with them. Follow-up telephone calls are strongly advised with these parents. The telephone conferences should effect some changes in the sets of these parents. We can also send printed information about stuttering to these parents to supplement our telephone conversations. This type of reference material has the advantage that the parent can turn to it at any time and read it. It also avoids many misunderstandings since, over time, people tend to forget or distort what they have heard. The letter about stuttering in Appendix B can be used here.

We have yet to address the most serious problem, parents who are disinterested to the point where they will not come in for a conference or parents who are angry about the stuttering and penalize the child when he stutters. A telephone conference may produce some positive results here, but I tend to be pessimistic. When confronted with this situation, I first try the telephone conference and, if not successful, follow up with the informational letter presented in Appendix B. We can only hope that these parents will listen to us and/or read the material. If they do this, there may be a change in their sets, perhaps even to the point where they will come in for a conference. In any event, we must attempt in some way to change the home environment and the only way to accomplish this is through the cognitive sets of the parents.

Still another way to achieve some change in the parents' cognitive sets is through record keeping. If the client is having success in controlling his speech, the parents should be made aware of the successes. You could have the client share his log book or record book with the parents or you might call them with periodic reports. If the parents see progress, their set may change to the point where they will come in for a conference. In the event that the client is making significant changes in his speech everywhere but in the home, you should explain this to the parents. There are two reasons for this. First, the parents are authority figures and all stutterers have difficulty in speaking to authority figures. Second, the client will have stuttered to his parents for many years and this form of speech is habituated in this environment.

There is no easy answer to dealing with parents who have a negative set to their child's stuttering. We must first of all attempt to change the cognitive sets through information about stuttering. If this has no effect, the only alternative for us is to attempt to work around their disruptive influence by providing the client a reward-oriented environment in the school and hope that this will offset the negative influence in the home. With older clients, we can also work with them in terms of understanding why their parents react to the stuttering as they do. We can point out to these clients that their parents are frustrated, just as they are, and they respond to their frustrations by becoming angry. Sometimes when a client understands the source of parental anger, it reduces its negative impact.

Parents Who Themselves Stutter

This unique situation calls for some special attention. If one of the client's parents is also a stutterer, it creates some rather serious problems in terms of the stuttering parent's cognitive set. In that the parent has experienced the penalties associated with stuttering, he will have a very special reason for not wanting his child to stutter. He will have a thorough, though subjective, understanding of his child's problem but he is also more emotionally involved in the problem than a nonstuttering parent would be. He will have more guilt associated with his child's stuttering, a feeling that he caused it because of his own stuttering. He may feel that his child stutters because the child imitated his stuttering. Because of his emotional involvement in the child's stuttering, he will have a tendency to overreact, making the problem more serious than it actually is and, in so doing, make the stuttering worse.

The parent who stutters must be carefully counseled in terms of the causes of stuttering. He must be made aware that imitation of stuttering does not cause a child to stutter. He must also be shown how he might have a tendency to overreact and counseled in terms of how to respond when his child does stutter. His cognitive set must be changed from one of guilt to one of acceptance of his child's stuttering. The major difficulty you will have in this situation is to get the parent to create *two* cognitive sets, one related to his own stuttering and the other related to his child's stuttering. The two will be different. Again, information about the phenomenon is the most useful tool we have to change the cognitive set and, who knows, you might even help the parent deal with his own stuttering problem.

Counseling centered on the five stages of grief is particularly important with the stuttering parent. The intensity of his feelings will be greater and he will need more reassurrance and support from the clinician. Again, allowing the parent to express his feelings of denial, anger, and depression will be a positive action. It will create no additional problems and may help him resolve some of the existing problems.

Chapter 6

Factors Influencing Therapy

THE CLIENT'S MOTIVATION

We cannot assume that all of our clients are interested in receiving therapy for their stuttering. While some clients seek therapy for their stuttering, others are sent to us for therapy. However, the effectiveness of our therapy is directly related to the motivation the client has to work on his stuttering. If a client seeks therapy for his stuttering, we can make the assumption that there is some approach motivation and by using appropriate rewards in our therapy we can strengthen and/or maintain the motivation.

Our problem is with the client who is SENT to us for therapy. With no motivation to work on the stuttering, we must attempt to create "artificial" approach motivation through our rewards. If our rewards are appropriate and strong, we can create approach motivation in the therapy environment. However, we will have to make further adjustments in our treatment program when it is time to generalize the new speech behaviors to environments where we no longer have direct control over the rewards. Since we face a unique clinical situation with each type of client, we will discuss each of these conditions, motivated clients and unmotivated clients, and consider the clinical influence of the client's attitude toward therapy.

Clients Seeking Therapy

These clients already have some approach motivation. We must now strengthen it as necessary and maintain it. This is possible through the rewards the client is provided. However, as the new speech behavior becomes more generalized and the speech more fluent, approach motivation wanes. The stuttering has been reduced in severity to the point where it no longer "hurts," it is now just an "annoyance." To maintain the motivation of the client we must find an appropriate reward to maintain the approach motivation or, perhaps, find a penalty which the client wants to avoid to create avoidance motivation. This provides us with two forms of motivation to use with the client.

We can also use the influence of the client's significant others, especially the parents of younger clients, to help maintain the approach and avoidance motivation. If the significant others are not available or cooperative we must turn to other means to maintain the motivation. Let us consider the two alternatives.

Cooperative significant others. When the significant others are cooperative we can use their assistance in several ways. Most important, we can now create a "support system." A support system consists of significant others who understand why the client is in therapy and support his efforts to deal with his stuttering. They provide both incentives and rewards for the client as well as moral support during his therapy. This calls for counseling the significant others in terms of what and when to reward and how to support the client. This type of assistance will increase the efficiency of our therapy.

Uncooperative or absent significant others. We now have a more difficult task in strengthening or maintaining the approach motivation since the only people involved are the clinician and the client. The client has no outside support system. To compensate for this we can attempt to enlist the assistance of other people in the client's environment such as other group members, teachers, counselors, or others in the school environment. If these people will provide understanding and support, the task of maintaining the motivation is easier. The rewards the client receives from these people are very important since they supplement the rewards that the client is receiving from us in therapy. If this type of support program is set up, it must have consistency and this must be coordinated by the clinician. These people can also be helpful if we turn to avoidance motivation but this should be done with caution. The use of penalty by untrained persons needs very close supervision. However, if done properly, the client's avoidance motivation can be an important factor in therapy.

Clients Sent for Therapy

These clients include both those children whose parents or teachers recommend therapy and also the adult stutterers who are referred for therapy but who do not actually want to enter therapy. Regardless of the reasons for their reluctance to enter therapy, it still means that they have no motivation to work on their speech. We have a problem in dealing with the unmotivated client. Our task is to create motivation since without it, our therapy will have little effect. We have very few alternatives. We may have limited success creating motivation by discussing the problem with the client but this can be applied only to older clients. In this highly cognitive approach we can discuss the problems that the client faces and how therapy can help. But, while the client is dealing with this on an intellectual level, his emotional level may be rejecting the logic because of fear of failure and other emotional factors. Discussions are an important part of creating motivation but we must supplement this with rewards that create approach motivation. The approach motivation we create this way may be artificial but, as long as the client learns new speech behavior that reduces the stuttering, the reasons he is learning are not important.

Again, as the new speech behavior become more effective and the stuttering becomes less of a problem, the approach motivation may fade. We may have to turn to avoidance motivation to maintain interest in therapy.

Cooperative significant others. With cooperation from the significant others we can create a strong support system; the unmotivated client needs all of the support and understanding that the significant others can provide. A strong reward program from the significant others can provide us with valuable assistance as we attempt to motivate the client for therapy. Again, the significant others must be carefully counseled. They must understand that the client has no interest in therapy. They must also understand how their assistance will help motivate the client. The significant others should be carefully supervised through reports and conferences. The clinician must be aware of what is happening with the client in the significant other's environment.

Uncooperative or absent significant others. This is the most difficult clinical task we will face. We are attempting to do therapy with a client who does not want to be in therapy and there are no significant others to help us create motivation. Artificial approach motivation can be created in the clinical environment through our rewards but, once the client leaves this environment, there is no one to maintain the motivation. We can again turn to the assistance of other group members, teachers, counselors, and others in the school environment but this only partially replaces the support system that the client needs. Again, this program must be supervised so that it has consistency. This clinical situation is not hopeless but our clinical skills are taxed to the utmost to motivate the client for therapy. This situation does not lead to the most effective therapy for the client. We can turn to avoidance motivation in the clinical environment but it will not be as effective with this client as with the others we have discussed. The use of avoidance motivation by others who might be assisting us should only be done with extreme care.

PEER PRESSURE

Peer pressure is a factor faced in the schools, regardless of the age of the client. The pressure only takes different forms between the early elementary ages and the late high school ages. It is probably at its peak somewhere between the 7th and 10th grades, depending on the individual child. Peer pressure can have a decidedly negative effect on therapy if the client feels that his peers disapprove of his receiving therapy. He may feel that he is considered "different" or "handicapped" when he is taken out of the classroom to go for therapy. This goes against the need to fit in with and to be accepted by the peer group.

If the client is teased about his stuttering by his peers in the school environment, it is devastating since he is in contact with this group of peers during all the time he is in school. He is in competition with these peers academically and socially and his stuttering interferes with this competition in both areas. His classroom performance will more than likely suffer because of his reluctance to speak in class. He is also handicapped as he attempts to compete socially. Having his stuttering brought to the fore by having to go for therapy only makes the problem worse. Clinical resistance is not an uncommon response to this situation. The clinician must deal with it the best she can. She can try to ignore it but it will not just go away.

Although we can not eliminate peer pressure in the school environment, we can attempt to minimize its negative impact. To do this we must attempt to change the client's cognitive set about himself and his stuttering. If the client has a poor self-image, he is especially susceptible to peer pressure. We might approach this by working on the list of assets discussed earlier, emphasizing his assets while minimizing the liabilities he feels he has. Through this we are attempting to increase the client's security in his dealings with his peers so that he can become more independent of their reactions to him. We can also attempt to reduce the impact of negative peer responses to the client's stuttering by discussing listener reactions to stuttering with him. This may help him understand why some of his peers react as they do when he stutters and this insight should reduce the effect of the negative reactions on him.

Group therapy offers us other means of dealing with negative peer pressure. In that the group members form their own peer group, the positive support of the group can be used to partially offset negative peer reactions the client may be encountering in school. If a group member is being subjected to severe negative peer pressure, the group could discuss the topic and the members share with the client their means of dealing with peer opinions and reactions. The group can be a powerful support system for the stuttering client whose peers are responding negatively to his stuttering or to his receiving therapy.

THE MATURITY OF THE CLIENT

When we talk about maturity, we are not necessarily talking about chronological age. We are talking about the cognitive and emotional maturity of the client. The more cognitive maturity we have with a client, the better we are able to teach the new concepts and speech behaviors we are working with. We are able to deal with these clients on a higher cognitive level and this accelerates learning.

The emotional maturity of the stuttering client is a matter of conjecture. As was mentioned earlier, the stutterer develops his negative emotional attitudes towards his stuttering at an early age and never outgrows them. Regardless of the age of the stutterer, he reacts to his stuttering much as he did at a much earlier age. It is still a frightening and demeaning factor in his life. He does not approach it from an adult point of view, accepting it and dealing with it in an unemotional way. This lack of emotional maturity will tend to offset to some degree his cognitive maturity. One way to view this is to recognize that there are two "personalities" associated with the stutterer: his intellectual, cognitive side and his emotional side. He may intellectually agree to work on a specific speech behavior but the emotional side, his fear of his speech, prevents him from following through.

THE CLIENT'S ATTENDING BEHAVIORS

For our therapy to be effective, the client must be attending to therapy. If he is attending to stimuli other than those provided by the clinician, his clinical learning will be diminished. As long as we have approach and/or avoidance motivation, we have the client's attention, since he is performing the behaviors that are rewarded and/or not producing the behaviors that result in penalty. However, if we lose the client's attention, we must deal with this directly. Our approach to this is shown in the CIM. In this situation the client is rewarded for attending behaviors and penalized for nonattending behaviors. As with any behavior, the reward will increase the occurrence of attending behaviors and penalty will decrease the occurrence of nonattending behaviors. Of course, this is all dependent on the appropriateness of the reward and the penalty. If the reward and penalty are appropriate, we should be able to regain the client's attention to therapy quickly. Once this is accomplished and the approach and/or avoidance motivation reinstated, we can shift our focus back to the speech behavior while continuing to monitor the client's attending behaviors.

CLINICAL RESISTANCE AND THE COGNITIVE SET

When a client is "forced" to have therapy for his stuttering, that is, his parents agree he may have therapy even though the client does not want it, we can understand his resisting our attempt to help him with his speech. His resistance may be due either to the fact that he really does not feel there is a need to change the speech or to a negative cognitive set, including a great deal of fear of the stuttering. But, what about the client who requests assistance and then resists all of our efforts to help him? What is the source of this clinical resistance? Why did he come to therapy if he is going to resist the treatment? He may appear stubborn or obstinate, but the source of the resistance is the fear of the stuttering, his negative cognitive set. We have here a conflict between the intellectual and the emotional sides of the stutterer. Intellectually he knows that he should do something about his speech and, therefore, he seeks help. However, the emotional side is resisting any attempt to change the stuttering. It is not that the stutterer enjoys his stuttering, but rather that he is "comfortable" with it. It is a predictable part of him. He knows this aspect of himself but he does not know what to expect if the stuttering is changed. He has adjusted his life style and expectations to his stuttering, establishing a compromise with his stuttering. In this way he has his life "in balance" and is afraid that therapy might disrupt the balance. Strange as it might sound, some stutterers prefer their "comfortable" stuttering to changing their speech into something unknown and unpredictable, something they do not "trust."

There is also the fear the stutterer has of attempting to change his stuttering. After all, he has tried to change it in the past and has failed. He does not need any more failures. In therapy, we are not only dealing with the intellectual side of the stutterer, we are also dealing with the stutterer's cognitive set, his emotional side, which has developed through years of stuttering. For most stutterers, it is easier to talk about the stuttering than to do something about it.

The clinical resistance can also take a very subtle form that misleads many clinicians. In this instance the client is very cooperative in the clinical environment but does not work on the speech outside the clinic room. This failure to work outside the clinical environment is from one of two major sources: clinical resistance due to a negative set (primarily fear) or because of lack of motivation to work on the speech. In either event, if we are going to extend the new speech behavior to other environments, we will have fo deal with the client's set and motivation.

Chapter 7

Group Therapy

THE SHAPING GROUP

Almost every speech clinician working in a school environment does "group therapy." There are probably as many forms of group therapy as there are clinicians. This condition exists because there are no references the clinician can turn to that set forth guidelines on how to do group therapy. So, each clinician creates her own form of working with a group of clients. Much of the group therapy practiced is really "therapy in a group," individual therapy provided in a group setting. In the school environment, this is partially due to the environmental role models of "teachers" and "students." The clients then play a passive role in therapy, just as they would in the classroom.

The term "group therapy" implies that there is therapeutic interaction between the members of the group, that the group members are involved in both providing therapy for other members of the group and receiving therapy from other group members. During the past 10 years a highly specialized form of group therapy, the shaping group, has been developed for the speech clinician, particularly for the clinician working in the school environment. The operational aspects of the shaping group are presented in this chapter. There is neither the time nor the space to give a detailed presentation of all aspects of the shaping group in this book. The reader is referred to the chapter, "The Shaping Group: Habituating New Behaviors in the Stutterer" (Leith, 1979) for a detailed presentation of this form of group therapy as applied directly to stuttering. More general discussions of the shaping group are also to be found in other books and articles by Leith (1982, 1984). In these references you will find that four different shaping groups are defined. In this book the types of shaping groups are reduced to three due to the unique population of stutterers the school clinician deals with.

CONTRASTS BETWEEN GROUP THERAPY FORMS

In the more traditional therapy in a group, as the clinician works with a member of the group, the other group members listen and watch the therapy as they are waiting their turn. All modeling, guidance, and information are provided by the speech clinician. She also evaluates all of the responses of the clients and administers the rewards and penalties. Interaction among group members is at a minimum. Learning occurs with each group member only when they are receiving therapy from the clinician.

By contrast, all members of the shaping group are actively involved in therapy at all times. The group members join in providing the modeling, guidance, and information for each other. Judgments of the responses and the application of either reward or penalty are also shared by the group members. All group members are expected to be both clinicians and clients. They act as clinicians when the group is focusing on another group member, and are clients when the group focuses on them. Since they are always involved in the therapeutic interaction, they are constantly involved in a learning experience.

LEARNING FUNCTIONS OF THE SHAPING GROUP

One of the most important things that a client must learn in therapy is to monitor his own speech. If he does not have this skill, there will be no carry-over of the new speech behavior to outside environments. The client must be aware of when and if the old speech behavior is occurring so that he can make the necessary corrections in order for the new speech behavior to occur. In more traditional group therapy where the clinician makes all of decisions regarding the correctness of the members' behaviors and administers the rewards and penalties, the members of the group have little opportunity to learn to monitor speech. The issue of listening skills is addressed only when the individual group member is receiving his therapy.

Shaping group members are expected not only to monitor their own speech, but also to monitor the speech of the other group members. They learn to monitor their own speech not only to achieve the rewards from the group but also to avoid group penalty. They monitor the speech of other members in order to apply either a reward or penalty. Self-monitoring skills are carefully taught in the shaping group. This makes the generalization of the new speech behavior to other environments much easier and faster.

The shaping group also provides its members with an opportunity to use their new speech behavior in a semisocial environment where the basic speech form is conversational. It might be viewed as a "half-way house" for the client who stutters. He can practice his new speech behavior with a group of people, talking on a variety of subjects. The group members will provide him with honest feedback in terms of how effective he is in using the new speech behavior.

The shaping group provides the opportunity to create "role playing," dealing with situations a group member may be having a particularly difficult time with. If a group member must give an oral report in class, the group can serve as the "class" while the client gives his oral report, using his new speech behavior. Other members of the group could use the group to "practice" talking to clerks in stores, ordering in restaurants, asking questions in class, and so forth. This aspect of the group function represents the gradual introduction of an S— where the S— is so strong that the client is unable to use his new speech behavior.

If we have a homogeneous group, a group made up of all stutterers, there can be sharing of attitudes, emotions, and feelings. The stutterer feels, and often rightfully so, that no one understands how he feels about his stuttering. This is true, except with another stutterer. There is much to be learned in this type of exchange in a group. Each member will have a slightly different view of the same problem and members should gain insight into their own attitudes, emotions, and feelings as they participate in such group discussions.

HOMOGENEOUS AND HETEROGENEOUS GROUPS

Groups where all members have the same type of communication disorder may be easier to deal with and, perhaps, a bit more efficient. In that all group members can focus on the same problem, the clinician's task is simpler. There are still other advantages. If a group consists of all stutterers, there will be a common bond since they have all experienced the effects of stuttering on their lives. This leads to a close interaction between the group members. Individual group members have a sense of belonging to the group since this is the only place where they can express their feelings and others will understand. They are working on the same speech behavior so they can assist on another in learning the behavior, strengthening it, and using it outside the group.

There is also a negative side when a group is made up of clients who all stutter. Just because a client stutters, it does not mean that he is comfortable around another person who stutters. I have found just the opposite. Many stutterers are more uncomfortable around another stutterer than a nonstutterer would be. Part of the reason for this is that when the stuttering occurs, it reminds the individual of his own problem, and he is often more embarrassed since he knows how embarrassed he is when he stutters. Finally, when the stutterer finds himself reacting negatively to another person's stuttering, he feels guilty. After all, this is what angers him, others reacting negatively to his stuttering. This attitude can inhibit group interaction since each group member wants to be "kind" to the other group members. There is a lack of objectivity about stuttering in a homogeneous group. If this problem does exist in a homogeneous group, the clinician can deal with it by explaining that feelings such as these are normal and that they will disappear as the members become involved in the group and with helping one another.

Groups that are made up of clients with a variety of disorders also have advantages and disadvantages. One advantage is that the stuttering client has an opportunity to use his new speech behavior with a group of peers who do not stutter, and this is more realistic than talking with a group of stutterers. He can share some of his feelings with people who can give him more objective feedback. Further, it gives the stutterer an opportunity to recognize that other people also have difficulty with their speech. This is an important factor since many stutterers feel that they are the only people who have a problem with their speech. The peer interactions in heterogeneous groups are more natural than in a homogeneous group of stutterers. Again, though, the heterogeneous group also has some disadvantages.

The client who stutters may not be willing to share his attitudes, emotions, and feelings with the heterogeneous group since the other members would not understand the problem. Another disadvantage concerns the problems the clinician has in dealing with a number of communication problems in the same group. Some of the problems will be complex, such as the stuttering, while others may not be as complex. The clinician must then govern how much time the group is spending on each group member's problem.

Another aspect of homogeneous and heterogeneous groups concerns how far along each member of the group is in therapy. If all members of the group, for example, are just beginning therapy, this is another form of a homogeneous group. This has the advantage that all members are in the initial stages of therapy, but this will demand some individual attention in the group. In a heterogeneous group where members are in different phases of therapy, those group members who are more advanced in therapy can assist the clinician in teaching new behaviors to group members just starting therapy. This is a good exercise for the more advanced group members and will help get the shaping group started sooner and easier.

In setting up a shaping group the clinician has two factors to consider when grouping, namely, the types of disorders of the potential members and how far along in therapy they are. There are no guidelines for selection but all combinations have both advantages and disadvantages. If a particular combination is awkward and creating problems for the clinician, she can shift members between her groups.

WHEN TO USE THE SHAPING GROUP

When we consider the three basic steps in therapy, getting the new behavior to occur, stabilizing the new behavior, and generalizing the new behavior, the shaping group is most effective in the last two steps. This does not mean that it can not be used in the first step, only that there will be a mixture of therapy in a group and shaping group during this step. If all of the clients who are to make up the shaping group are new clients, the clinician will have to do some individual therapy with each client until their new behavior is beginning to occur. The process can then shift to the shaping group. If only one new client is introduced to an on-going shaping group, a variation in group organization, discussed later in the chapter, will allow this client to receive individual attention without disrupting the on-going group. Each speech clinician will determine when the shaping group works best for her, considering the number of clients she is working with, her time schedule, and other factors.

THE CLINICIAN'S ROLE AS SHAPING GROUP LEADER

The role of shaping group leader involves activities quite different from those the clinician performs in therapy in a group. She is no longer a "clinician" in the strictest sense of the word in that she is not involved in the direct provision of therapy. She is now involved in training the members of the group to function as clinicians, for themselves and the other group members. This training is accomplished through modeling, guidance, and information provided by the speech clinician. She is adhering to the CIM model since she is still teaching. However, she is now teaching behaviors other than speech behaviors. As the group members learn to function as "clinicians" in the shaping group, the clinician withdraws her stimuli (modeling, guidance, and information) and assumes a different role. With the group members maintaining the therapeutic interaction of the group, the clinician can now become more of an observer, a moderator, an orchestrator. She continues to carefully monitor the group interaction and therapy, only intervening when necessary. Her role is more passive than active and the majority of talking is done by the group members rather than the clinician. For many clinicians, this has proven to be the most difficult aspect of assuming the role of shaping group leader, to be quiet and not monopolize the group interaction. It is foreign to us to allow the clients to perform their own therapy, even under our strict guidance. However, it does work— more effectively in many cases since the clients usually demand more of themselves than does the clinician.

TYPES OF SHAPING GROUPS

To accommodate for age differences in groups, three levels of shaping groups have been established. Each group level is unique in that the clients at each level have different needs, social maturity, and cognitive maturity. The three levels of groups are the elementary shaping group, the junior shaping group, and the senior/adult shaping group.

Elementary Shaping Group

Typically, children between the ages of 5 and 11 make up this group. Further, a 3-year age range among the group members should be maintained. The size of the group should be limited, if possible, to three children, since children of this age lack the social maturity to interact with larger groups. The male/female ratio in the younger groups is not important but does begin to affect the group interaction at the upper end of the age range. These are only guidelines, not hard-and-fast rules. The maturity of each client is a factor the clinician must consider when assigning clients to groups.

Junior Shaping Group

We are now dealing with children between the ages of 12 and 15. Due to increased social maturity, the group can function with four members with a 4-year range of ages between group members. The clinician must keep in mind that she is now dealing with clients who are entering the strange age of puberty. This is going to have a direct effect on the age range of the group, the group size, and the male/female ratio, which now becomes an important factor. Decisions about the makeup of the group must be made by the clinician who is involved with the group. In making the decisions she must consider the clients' ages, their degree of social maturity, and how they relate to the opposite sex. There must be careful planning with this group and the clinician will find her role as group leader a bit more complicated. This is a sensitive age for the clients and group interactions may tend to be a bit more difficult to initiate and control.

Senior/Adult Shaping Group

The ages of clients involved in this group are somewhat dependent on the local rules governing who is eligible for clinical services. We will base our group on the upper limit of 24 years of age. Therefore, this group may consist of clients between the ages of 16 and 24. With this wide an age span, we would want to limit the range of ages within a group to no more than 4 years. We also attempt to limit the size of the group to four members. The male/female ratio is not as important with this shaping group but the clinician will have to make some decisions in this regard according to the maturity of the clients. If the clinician has a mature group of clients, the group size can be increased to five.

ACTIVITIES OF GROUP MEMBERS

The Clients

The shaping group can not operate efficiently unless all group members participate in the group interaction. This involves the monitoring of the speech behaviors of other group members, administering rewards or penalties, and participating in group discussions. Regardless of whether the group is homogeneous or heterogeneous, the members of the group must know what behaviors all other members are working on and, if they are to reward or penalize behavioral performances, how well the behaviors can be performed. This information is provided during the formation of the group as the clinician identifies each group member and what behavior they are working on. If some group members are more advanced in therapy, they can demonstrate their new behaviors. Members who are just starting therapy will probably have to receive individual attention in the group until the new behavior is beginning to occur. This will help identify the new behavior for the other members of the group. The group members can then become involved in shaping the behavior to the behavior change goal.

This process of identification of behavior change goals forms the basis of improving listening skills since the group members must then listen to and identify a variety of speech behaviors. The clients are being taught to listen to both *what* is said and *how* it is said. All of this is fundamental to self-monitoring and this is the basic skill needed for carry-over of the new speech behaviors to other speaking environments. As the monitoring skills improve, so will the speech performance of the group members.

The group leader will have to specifically train the group members to administer rewards and penalties. This is a new behavior for them. They can be taught this new behavior through information provided by the group leader as well as through the modeling provided by both the group leader and other members of the group. The most important source of modeling will be the group leader and she should explain both what she is doing and why she is doing it. It is extremely important that the group leader explain that group members can help one another through rewards and penalties. The reward concept will not be difficult to explain but penalty will offer some challenges. I have found it helpful to explain this in terms of "feedback." A group member can not change a behavior if he is not aware of when he is performing it incorrectly. The member needs both types of feedback, rewards when he does it correctly and penalty when he does it incorrectly. Again, the penalty we are talking about is not severe. It is more in the form of letting the person know that what they did was not correct or acceptable.

In that all members of the shaping group are involved in administering both rewards and penalties, these contingent events are quite strong. The shaping group members make up a "peer" group and this takes on added significance when rewards or penalties are administered. Since the group members are operating in peer social interaction, they have strong approach motivation to receive rewards from their peers. There is also a strong avoidance motivation to avoid being penalized by their peer group.

Because we are dealing with clients who stutter, it is all the more important that they participate in group interactions and discussions. First of all, this provides them with an opportunity to practice their new speech behavior in a conversational mode. Secondly, as the topic of conversation changes, it provides the client with an opportunity to use his new speech behavior while talking about a variety of subjects, some more emotional than others.

The Clinician

The role of group leader calls for some new behaviors on the part of the clinician. She is no longer a clinician working in an individual therapy setting. She is now guiding a therapeutic interaction, acting as a moderator when the need arises. She is more of a supervisor than an active clinician. Let us examine some of the tasks the group leader must assume.

The clinician models:

1. The administration of rewards
2. The administration of penalty
3. The performance of new speech behaviors for new group members
4. The various tasks that make up the role of the group leader
5. The participation and interaction in group activities.

The clinician provides guidance for:

1. The group members in determining rewards and penalties to be administered in the group
2. The group interaction to prevent it from drifting away from therapy
3. The group interaction to maintain a balance of rewards and penalties so the group does not become either too positive or too negative
4. The group interaction so that no member receives too much penalty
5. The group requirements for behavioral performance for rewards so that they are within the member's capabilities.

The clinician provides information about:
1. The individual group member's behavior change goals
2. The operational rules for the shaping group
3. The purpose of applying rewards and/or penalties to other members of the group.

OPERATING THE SHAPING GROUP

Instructions

The first step in creating a shaping group is to set forth the rules and regulations of the group. All members of the group must understand how the group will operate and what they are expected to do as a member of the group. The clinician should stress the fact that all members must participate in the group interactions. Included in this information are the reasons for using rewards and penalties. It would be advisable to discuss this with the group members after the information has been presented to make sure that everyone understood what they had been told.

Identification of Behavior Change Goals

With any type of heterogeneous or homogeneous group, the clinician should identify the behavior change goal of each group member and describe or, if possible, have the group member demonstrate their proficiency with the new behavior. All behavior change goals should be clearly understood by the group members before proceeding. A group discussion of behavior change goals would be in order here. This is an essential part of starting the shaping group since the effectiveness of the group is dependent on the application of rewards and penalties to the appropriate behaviors.

Rewards and Penalties

Before the group interaction can begin, a decision must be made as to what will be used as a reward and as a penalty. The same reward and penalty must be used for all group members. The group leader and the group members must decide on what would be rewarding and what would be penalizing. Verification of the reward and penalty will be made by the group leader in observing the effects of the rewards and penalties on the behaviors once the group commences. The group leader should not decide on the reward and the penalty without input from the group members. Some guidelines for selecting the reward and penalty would include such factors as ease of application, not too time consuming, and not disruptive of the group interaction. A token economy will satisfy all of these requirements and there will be no problem with the actual reward since there can be a variety of backup rewards for the group members to select from.

If other forms of rewards and penalties are used, consider that with visual events, the recipient must be looking at the individual applying a reward to be aware of it. This is quite difficult in a group situation. However, one group waved small white flags for reward and red flags for penalty and it worked very well. Auditory signals seem better adapted to this type of clinical interaction. The auditory signals probably should not be verbal phrases such as, "That was good" or "That was not very good." If presented during a group interaction, they interrupt the therapy. A group might consider such things as a hand clap for reward and a finger snap for penalty. Other things to be considered are a cough, clearing the throat, a tongue click, the words "yes" and "no," and various noise makers. The danger here is that the noise level of reward or penalty can interfere with the group activities.

Getting the Group Started

The group interaction can begin after the instructions are given, group members' behaviors identified, and the reward and penalty determined. We will discuss a particular group since there are so many possible combinations: types of shaping groups and types of homogeneous or heterogeneous groups. We will discuss an elementary shaping group made up of clients with a variety of disorders. Each client can produce their new speech behavior on a more or less regular basis. The stutterer in the group is working on easy talking. All members of the group are still dependent on the reward for the speech performance. The group will be reward oriented as it begins. The group is started by having the members discuss a neutral but interesting topic, such as vacations or hobbies. Each member is asked to make a comment on the topic. As each member speaks, the clinician might provide some form of guidance to prompt the new behaviors. With the stutterer, she might give a gesture which indicates "talk with your lips." When the stutterer speaks, using his easy talking, she rewards him for his new speech behavior, modeling the giving of a reward for the other group members. She continues to model rewarding new speech behaviors, encouraging other group members to join her. When a group member rewards another member for a new behavior, she rewards him for his new rewarding behavior. She is rewarding the member for his monitoring and rewarding of another group member's speech. She wants to encourage members to reward one another, so the rewarding behavior is itself rewarded when it occurs. The group process is operational when the group members begin to reward each other for their new speech behavior. At this time the clinician fades her modeling, allowing the group members to provide their own modeling. The clinician then assumes the role of group leader, monitoring and guiding.

Penalty should not be introduced into the group until the group process is stable, with all members participating in the discussions and rewarding each other. Penalty is particularly useful as the group members become more engrossed in the discussion topics. They become more interested in *what* they are saying as opposed to *how* they are saying it. They then tend to "forget" their new speech behavior. For example, the stutterer becomes so involved in telling about his vacation that he forgets to do his easy talking. Another member catches this and penalizes the stutterer, perhaps by removing a token. This reminds the stutterer to use his easy talking. At the same time, the clinician rewards the group member for catching the stutterer doing hard talking. This is another monitoring behavior the clinician wants to encourage so it is rewarded. It is extremely important to remember than an incorrect behavior is only penalized when we are certain that the client can produce the correct behavior.

VARIATIONS IN GROUP ORGANIZATION

When the group is stable and operating effectively, group members should be trained to act as group leader. The clinician has provided the model of the group leader and she now allows a group member to lead the group while she provides guidance. The clinician can then fade her group leader role and assume other roles. When group members can assume the group leader role, the clinician is free to organize the group in several different ways.

With a group where a member needs individual attention or a new member who is just starting therapy is being added, the group can continue to operate with a member group leader while the clinician provides the individual therapy. The group should not continue under the direction of a member group leader over an extended period of time.

From time to time the clinician should withdraw from all group interaction and observe the shaping group in operation. These "objective" observations are important so that both individual members and group interactions can be carefully observed. The clinician is free to do this if she has trained a group member to lead the group while she observes. This gives her the opportunity to evaluate the progress of each group member, make changes in the group organization if warranted, and determine if the group is working toward the proper goals of therapy.

In the event that it is impossible to limit the group size to that recommended here, there is still another variation to the shaping group that will solve this problem. If there is an elementary shaping group with six members, there are too many members for the group to operate effectively. In this instance the clinician selects three group members to form a shaping group. The other members are then assigned to serve as individual monitors to the three members of the shaping group. The monitors sit behind their "clients" and monitor their speech. Their job is to remind their "client" to use his new speech behavior when he enters the group discussion. They also provide rewards and penalties to their "clients." Although not directly involved in the group interaction, the monitors practice their listening skills as they monitor their "client's" speech. When the roles are reversed among the members of the shaping group, the additional practice in listening skills will be manifested in more consistent use of the client's new behaviors. By using group members as monitors, all members of the group are still involved in therapy and not waiting for their turn.

ADDING NEW MEMBERS TO A GROUP

A shaping group that is started at the beginning of the school year is an on-going clinical procedure. As members achieve their behavior change goal and are dismissed from therapy, new members are added. New members need to be introduced to the operational guidelines of the group, the behavior change goals of the various group members, and the reward and penalty system and the reasons for using them. The remaining group members should provide this information under the guidance of the clinician. This is a good review for the remaining members. All of this information can be presented in one meeting of the group. As the group resumes therapy, the new member learns to function as a group member through the modeling and guidance provided by the other group members. In this way, new members can constantly be added to an ongoing group.

THE CIM AND THE SHAPING GROUP

You should recognize that the CIM is the basis of the shaping group interactions. However, the stimulus now comes from a member of the group, perhaps in the form of a question. The member to whom the question was directed will think about it and then respond. This member's response is the stimulus for the group to evaluate and respond to. The reward and/or the penalty is very strong both because it comes from a peer group and because of the number of peers involved in administering it. The strength of the reward and/or penalty may vary from application to application. If there are three members of the group evaluating a response, they may not all agree that it should be rewarded or penalized. If only one member provides the reward, the reward is not very strong while a reward from two group members is stronger. A reward from all three members is the strongest and is usually applied to the most obviously correct response. This concept of strength of group reaction also applies to the application of a penalty.

An important task of the group leader during group interactions is to monitor the attending behaviors of the group members. If a group member's attention is waning, the clinician can focus the group on his attending behaviors for rewards or penalties.

Another very important clinical feature of the shaping group is that all group members assume specific stimulus roles. As they present rewards they become an S+ for the other group members. The S- role stems from applying penalty. These special stimulus roles are carried over outside the clinical environment. This means that when group members encounter each other in the school, they will "cue up" the correct behaviors and discourage the incorrect behaviors. This important function of the shaping group is a great aid in generalizing the new behaviors to other environments in the school.

Section II: Stuttering Therapy

In each treatment program an attempt was made to provide enough basic information on various clinical concepts so that you can proceed with therapy without having to look back in the book to refresh your memory. If additional information is needed, the page numbers enclosed in brackets refer you to the section of the book where the concept was discussed in detail.

Chapter 8

Cognitive Behavior Stuttering Therapy: An Overview

THE GOALS AND RATIONALE OF THERAPY

Our therapy program is not attempting to "cure" stuttering. Rather, our clinical goal is to teach the client a new speech behavior which, when used, results in speech that listeners would judge as "normal." With the older client we refer to this speech as *controlled fluency*. We will eliminate as much of the stuttering as we can through the new speech behavior and then teach the client techniques to deal with any stuttering blocks that might occur in such a way that they do not disrupt the "normal" flow of speech. With younger clients we use the term *easy talking* to describe the new speech behavior.

Our therapy is cognitive in nature since we will not only explain carefully to the older client all he wanted to know about stuttering but was afraid to ask, but also because we expect the client to learn to perform the new speech behavior and control techniques voluntarily when they are needed. He is to monitor his speech and apply the controls in greater or lesser degrees depending on the quality of his speech production in various speaking situations.

We will be training the client to be his own clinician. He will be trained to monitor his speaking environments, be aware of his emotional reactions to them, and then use the necessary controls to maintain "normal" speech in each situation. He will also be trained to maintain his new speech behavior after therapy has been terminated.

The therapy program is designed to deal with both the STUTTERER and the STUTTERING, even those clients with other handicaps such as learning disabilities or mental retardation. Special adjustments in the therapy program for these clients are discussed in Appendix C.

Our work with the stutterer will include changing his cognitive set and preparing him to be his own clinician. The work on the stuttering will be to reduce the frequency, intensity, and duration of stuttering blocks to the point where the stuttering is no longer a problem in the client's life; we can not "cure" the stuttering, we can only reduce the severity of stuttering to its lowest point. Our clients will continue to be stutterers but, for all intents and purposes, they would be considered normal speakers in all of their speaking situations.

We view the stuttering and the client as inseparable. The stuttering is not something "outside" the client, a "thing" that is happening to him. The client and the stuttering are one and the same. The stuttering affects the client's cognitive set and the cognitive set affects the stuttering. It is a vicious cycle that we must interrupt and change from the negative influence of the stuttering to a positive one for the controlled fluency. This is our clinical challenge. This interaction between the stuttering and the cognitive set before therapy is shown in the diagram below.

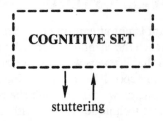

This diagram illustrates the interaction between the client's cognitive set and the stuttering before therapy. As the stuttering becomes more severe, it negatively influences the development of the cognitive set. And, as the cognitive set becomes more negative and fear of speaking becomes a major cognitive issue, the stuttering becomes more severe. It is during this time the stutterer develops two fears associated with his stuttering. He not only develops the fear that he will stutter, he also develops a fear associated with the duration of the stuttering block when it occurs. Basic to both fears is the feeling on the part of the client that he will appear "foolish" to his listener if he stutters or if the stuttering block lasts for a long period of time. Let us now go through the various steps in our stuttering therapy.

EVALUATION AND PLANNING PROCESS

Initial Evaluation and Planning

In our evaluation of the individual, our first task, after receiving permission from the parent to perform the evaluation, is to determine if the person is truly a stutterer. We determine this by careful observation of his speech during an interview. We test his speech in conversation, story telling (narration), and, if possible, reading aloud. We test these three forms of communication since each presents a different speech format to the client. A person may be able to conceal his stuttering in conversation and narration by substituting words. However, this is not possible in reading and this may be the only place where the stuttering becomes apparent and shows its true form. Having determined that the individual is a stutterer, we would administer either a formal or informal severity scale and gather other information about the stuttering, such as where it occurs in the speech, what speaking situations seem to precipitate it, and so forth. We would then determine a therapy goal which would be controlled fluency in our therapy approach. Our final task at this stage would be to formulate a therapy plan of how we would achieve our goal.

The Individual Education Planning Conference

We now present our findings and recommendations to the client's parent(s) at the individualized educational planning (IEP) conference. We present the results of our examination and set forth the therapy plan which we prepared after determining that the client was a stutterer. After discussing the therapy plan with the parents, they decide whether or not their child may receive therapy for the stuttering problem. Assuming that the parents agree to the therapeutic plan, we proceed to the next step of this pretreatment phase.

Informational Meeting with Client

Before we start into the actual treatment of the stuttering, we want to meet with the more mature client and give him some insight into his problem. We provide him with information about stuttering: what it is, where it occurs, and why it occurs. We will also set forth our therapy program and our goal. This information will reduce some of the fear of stuttering and make our therapy much easier since the client now knows what is happening to him when he stutters and where we are going in therapy. We are now ready to start the actual treatment of the stuttering.

CLINICAL PROCESS

Getting the New Behavior to Occur

The first step in therapy is shown in the following diagram. It is at this point that we change the interaction between the stuttering and the client's cognitive set. In all diagrams to follow, the primary focus of therapy is indicated by a solid line while the secondary focus is shown by a broken line.

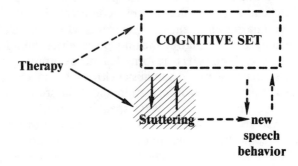

As noted in the diagram, the focus of therapy is on the establishment of the new speech behavior through modeling, guidance, and information from the clinician or through the use of a delayed auditory feedback (DAF) if one is available. Our influence on the client's cognitive set is almost incidental as we reward the occurrences of the new speech behavior. The new behavior, as it occurs, will reduce the amount of stuttering and effect positive changes in the client's cognitive set. Both of these factors then increase the quality of the new speech behavior as the fear level of the client is reduced and self-confidence is increased.

During this step in therapy we shift our stimulus role from an S0, a neutral stimulus, to an S+ by rewarding occurrences of the new speech behavior. The S- role for stuttering behavior is introduced toward the end of this step after the new behavior is beginning to occur more regularly.

Stabilizing the New Speech in the Clinical Environment

The next diagram shows the shifting emphasis of therapy. The focal point of therapy is now on stabilizing the new behavior that the client has learned to produce in the clinical environment.

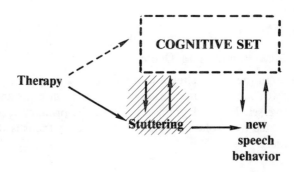

The therapy is now focused on stabilizing the new speech behavior so that the client is able to speak on any topic without reverting back to his old speech behavior, stuttering. The negative influence of the stuttering on the client's cognitive set has been removed and the positive influence of the new speech behavior is increased. Again, as the fears decrease and the self-confidence increases, the proficiency of the new speech behavior is increased. The rewards are gradually removed through an intermittent reward schedule to test the habituation of the new speech behavior and the resultant controlled fluency or easy talking. If the new speech behavior begins to falter as the rewards are withdrawn, the rewards must be increased to maintain the behaviors until they become more stable.

We maintain our roles of S+ and S−, although the S− role is rarely used since the new speech behavior is occurring consistently in the clinical environment.

Generalizing the New Speech Behaviors

As is indicated in the next diagram, the focus of therapy shifts again as the new speech behavior is introduced to outside environments. The emphasis is now on changing the client's cognitive set, which will in turn strengthen the new speech behavior.

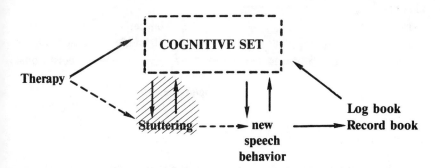

Once the new speech behavior is occurring consistently in the therapy room, it must be introduced to speaking situations outside the clinical environment. The client is instructed to use a log book to record information about his practice in using his new speech behavior in outside talking situations. Clients who cannot write keep a record book of their use of their new speech behavior by using a symbol system while, with very young clients, the parents keep a record book of their child's use of the new speech behavior.

Information contained in the log book (record book) is discussed in detail by the clinician and the client. We dwell on the successes the client has had with the new speech behavior. We use the log book as a means of changing the client's cognitive set. As the self-confidence increases, so does the proficiency of the new speech behavior. And, as the client experiences more success in talking situations, his fear of speaking is reduced. With older clients we are directly involved in training them to be their own clinician, able to recognize their successes, use their new-found confidence to introduce the new speech behavior into other speaking situations, and solve any speaking problems which might arise.

Maintenance of Controlled Fluency

When the new speech is occurring in all speaking situations and the stuttering is no longer a problem in the client's life, the responsibility of maintaining the speech is shifted to the client. This change in clinical strategy is shown below.

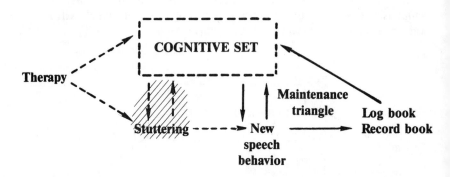

The client assumes more and more of the responsibility of evaluating his performance of his new speech behavior and maintaining his new set. The solid lines represent the relationships between the client's cognitive set, his controlled fluency, and the log book. The client is acting as his own clinician, while we monitor his performance as a clinician. We gradually fade our clinical input and contacts with the client as he demonstrates his ability to act as his own clinician.

When we have withdrawn all clinical contacts from the client, the therapy program is continued by the client. This is represented in the diagram by the solid lines which form the "maintenance triangle." To maintain his newly learned speech behavior, the client must continue to practice the behaviors on a regular basis, perhaps one practice per day, and enter them in his log book. As with any motor skill, such as playing the piano, the client must first practice to learn his new behavior and then practice to maintain it. If there is no practice, the performance level of the new skill will deteriorate, as will the proficiency level of the controlled fluency or easy talking.

Chapter 9

Treatment:
Ages 2 Through 8

This treatment program is designed for clients from 2 to 8 years of age. It takes into consideration and adjusts for the cognitive level of the client and his lack of writing skills. In this program we do not consider the stuttering and the new method of speech we will be teaching as being made up of several interrelated behaviors. Rather, we present the concept of stuttering as *hard talking* and the new method of speaking as *easy talking*. The clinical focus is on the single behavior event, the end result, rather than on the verbal behaviors which constitute the event since children of this age cannot comprehend the complexities of a number of behaviors interacting to produce a new way of talking.

Due to the cognitive level and lack of maturity of children in this age group, the treatment program is quite dependent on the cooperation of the parents and a home program. Both of these are especially important when working with a preschool child.

Some of the older clients in this age group may have the maturity and writing skills needed for the program for clients aged 9 through adult. You will have to make this decision based on your evaluation of the child, how the child fits into your clinical schedule, the treatment program used with other stutterers in his treatment group, and other such factors.

FACTORS INFLUENCING THIS THERAPY PROGRAM

Because of the range of ages of clients you will use this program with, there are some important factors that will influence your therapy. Take these into consideration as you adapt the treatment program to the individual client and to your clinical environment.

Client Motivation [71–75]

The motivation for therapy will vary according to the age and maturity of the client. Some children in this age group will recognize their problem and express their concern to their parents. These children come to therapy with some basic motivation. However, other children are sent to therapy because of their parent's concern or the concern of teachers and the speech clinician. In this instance the child comes to therapy with no motivation to work on his speech. Motivation is an important part of the effectiveness of your therapy so you will have to create motivation for the unmotivated client.

Peer Pressure [50, 74]

The basic need to be accepted by peers is present even in the very young child. When he is teased about his stuttering by his peers, this not only creates negative attitudes toward his speech, but also toward himself and his relationships with his peers. Leaving a classroom for therapy may be a major source of peer teasing and could produce a negative attitude toward therapy. You may find some clinical resistance on the part of the child because of this pressure. The peer pressure faced by children of this age is not as severe as with older children but it is still a factor you should be aware of.

Parent Influence—Home Program [71–75]

The parents are a major influence in the life of the child at this age. For this reason, we need their cooperation in the treatment program. This is particularly true with the preschool-aged child. Although it is possible to do therapy with the young stutterer without parental involvement, the effectiveness of the program will be seriously handicapped. It behooves you to encourage parent involvement in the therapy by having them carry on a home program. If there is no possibility of providing the child with a home program, it will be necessary to adjust the therapy program to compensate for this lack of support by enlisting the help of significant others in the client's life.

The Therapy Program

In that you are providing clinical services in the school environment, there are specific procedures and protocols which are dictated for you through federal regulations, specifically Public Law 94-142. A quick reference guide to these procedures and protocols is provided for you in Appendix D. The implementation of the following treatment program will be influenced by these regulations, and different states and districts have additional rules and regulations. Modify the following treatment program according to your district's regulations.

EVALUATION

THE STUTTERING

Assessment of the Speech

The first step in the evaluation is to determine if the child is actually stuttering or is only displaying normal dysfluencies [38]. You should focus on the child's emotional involvement in the speech dysfluencies which will be manifested by noticeable body tension, excessive body movement, secondary mannerisms, struggle behavior, and other behaviors not usually associated with normal speech dysfluencies in the speech of children of this age. If the child is reacting emotionally to the dysfluencies and manifesting some of these behaviors, we will consider him a stutterer. The severity of the child's stuttering is not a factor here. First, you must determine if the child is stuttering, and then determine the severity.

Having determined that the child is stuttering, evaluate the speech using either a formal or informal stuttering evaluation procedure (severity scales) [34]. This evaluation will give you both an indication of the severity of stuttering and a detailed account of the stuttering behaviors before therapy. This will provide you with a means of measuring your clinical progress.

When talking with the client do not use the term "stuttering." Ask him what his speech problem is. If he tells you that it is stuttering, introduce him to the term "hard talking." If the client says things like the words get stuck or he just cannot say words, tell him that you are going to call it hard talking since he has to work very hard to get the words out.

Descriptions of Secondary Mannerisms [36-37]

If you use an informal scale, be sure to include information about the secondary mannerisms such as how often the behavior is used, how intense or strong the behavior is when it occurs, and how long the behavior lasts once it occurs. For example, if the client blinks his eyes during a block, your description might be as follows: eye blinks occur immediately after the block starts and four or five blinks occur during the block.

Because of the ages of these children, the stuttering will not be as complex as that of older stutterers. There will be fewer secondary mannerisms and those that do exist will not be as complicated as with older stutterers.

—NOTES—

Speech Samples [34, 96]

You should evaluate the client's speech under two conditions: conversation and story telling. Conversational speech tests the speech under spontaneous conditions while story telling tests the speech under conditions of thinking/talking or propositionality.

THE STUTTERER

In addition to the direct evaluation of the stuttering, you will want to learn about the client's attitudes, emotions, and feelings [55–56]. You need to know how he views his stuttering and himself. Do not assume that if his stuttering appears rather mild to you, the listener, that the client will have a mild reaction to it.

Determine Attitudes About:

The stuttering [50–53]. In determining how the client feels about his stuttering, you will have to be subtle in your approach. Some questions you might ask your client are listed below but you should add questions according to your particular client. Try to avoid asking questions that can be answered in a single word.

Why do you think you talk hard?

What do you do when you talk hard?

Do you get angry with yourself when you talk hard?

Do you become frightened when you talk hard?

What do other people do when you talk hard?

The parent's responses [50, 65–67, 69]. It is important to determine the parents' response to the younger client when he stutters. Ask the client what his parents do when he stutters. You may find that each parent responds differently. This information might give you insight into factors that could be maintaining the stuttering. You may also gain some insight into problems you will have to deal with when you meet the parents at the conference. Some questions you might ask are:

What does your mother do when you talk hard?

What does your father do when you talk hard?

What has your mother or father said to you about your hard talking?

Peer responses [50, 74]. The need for peer acceptance is present even with children this age. Because the client spends a good share of his time in school with his peers, you should determine how the client feels his peers react when he stutters. This is especially important with clients in this group who regularly attend some form of preschool program or are in the classroom, interacting with their peers. Peer pressure is a factor you will have to deal with in therapy. You might ask:

How do the boys in your school act when you talk hard?

How do the girls in your school act when you talk hard?

Do the other children do or say anything to you when you talk hard?

Responses of "others" [50, 53]. Your client will also have opinions about how his listeners in general react to his stuttering. The older clients in this age group will have more social experiences with their stuttering so they should be able to give you more information than the younger clients. The client's interpretation of others' responses is important to you as you determine his overall attitude toward his stuttering. Some questions you could ask are:

What do people do when you talk hard?

What do people think when you talk hard?

What does your teacher do when you talk hard?

The client's responses [50–53]. You should determine what the client does when his listener reacts to his stuttering. How does he feel and what does he do when his listener reacts to his stuttering? Younger children in this age group may not be able to respond to these questions. A few of the questions you might ask are:

What do you do or think when your listener smiles when you talk hard?

What do you do or think when your listener frowns when you talk hard?

What do you do when other children tease you about your hard talking?

The client's self-concept [49–50]. On a more general level, you need to determine what the client thinks of himself. You will be determining the effect of the stuttering on his self-concept. The self-concept of the younger children in this age group may not have yet been affected. Older children may have experienced repeated failures in trying to modify their stuttering and this may be evident in their self-concept. Some questions you might ask are:

What are all the things about you that you like?

What is there about you that you do not like?

Previous therapy [51–54]. Your older client in this age group may have had treatment for his stuttering from other clinicians. It is important for you to find out what type of therapy he has had. If he has a negative attitude toward his previous therapy, you may have to work with his attitude before starting your own therapy. You also need to know what procedures previous clinicians used with the client. You may find yourself repeating procedures other clinicians have used and that the client has a negative attitude toward. You should ask the following questions:

What other therapy have you had for your hard talking?
What kinds of things did you do in therapy?
How did your therapy help you with your speech?
Are you still able to use some of the things you learned in therapy?

Observations and Judgments to Make

In addition to asking questions, you can learn a great deal about your client by observing him during your evaluation. Some of the more important things for you to observe include the client's verbal level, his assertiveness, and sensitive areas in his life.

Verbal/nonverbal. How verbal is the client? If the client is reacting to his stuttering by withdrawing he will be relatively nonverbal. He will answer questions in the shortest way possible and will rarely volunteer speech. Other clients will be very verbal even though they are quite severe stutterers. This will give you some insight into how the client copes with his stuttering and this attitude will influence your therapy.

Assertive/nonassertive. Most typically, you will find the stutterer withdrawn and nonassertive. This client may speak softly and be quite nonverbal. He may also rarely look at you when speaking. On the other hand, there are some stutterers who are quite assertive in spite of their stuttering. They are outgoing, speak up, are verbal, and maintain eye contact with you even while they are stuttering. However, beware of making a judgment here based solely on eye contact. There are cultures where direct eye contact is interpreted as an act of hostility and children influenced by these cultures will not maintain eye contact [53]. The client's assertiveness will have a significant influence on your therapy. Assertive clients will be more willing to use easy talking outside the clinical environment.

Sensitive issues. There will probably be sensitive topics or issues for the client which, when discussed, create more stuttering. You should determine these topics or issues in order to avoid them in early therapy and to use them to test his control over his speech later in therapy. Issues you should check into are (a) peer relationships; (b) relationships with the opposite sex; (c) interaction with parents; (d) school environment.

General adjustment. The overall adjustment of the client should also be considered. You should attempt to determine how the client has adjusted to his environment. You will have to check with the parents and teachers to gather this information. Investigate the following areas:

(1) relations with peers, male and female
(2) classroom behavior
   (a) class clown
   (b) behavior problems
   (c) withdrawn
(3) home environment.

CONFERENCE WITH PARENTS

PRESENT PROBLEM TO PARENTS

When you discuss your findings with the parents in the IEP Conference, it is important to remember that the parents do not understand the complexities of stuttering and, further, are emotionally involved with their child [65]. Avoid the use of professional jargon and use terms that the parent will understand. One of the most difficult factors you will have to present to the parents is the client's emotional reaction to his stuttering [49–54]. Make sure that the parents have a basic understanding of the problem and how you plan to treat it [95–101]. With children in this age group, discuss the influence the home environment will have on your therapy. Delay asking the parents if they would be willing to assist in the treatment program until after they have approved of your therapy program. If the parents agree that their child may receive therapy, you should get as much information from them as possible to assist you with your therapy.

AREAS TO EXPLORE WITH PARENTS

1. You should determine the parents' feelings as to why their child stutters [38, 65]. This may be the source of much anxiety in the home, and of parental negative reactions to the child.

2. Ask the parents how they respond to the child when he stutters. There are only three possible responses: to reward the client by being solicitous, to penalize the client by a negative reaction, or to ignore the stuttering [65]. The last response will be very rare since most parents will have some sort of overt response to their child's stuttering.

3. Another important area of questioning concerns the reactions of siblings when the child stutters [50]. Your questions should include both younger and older siblings.

4. Playmates are a peer group for the child and you should discuss this with the parents. Ask the parents how playmates react when the child stutters [50].

5. The home environment should be carefully examined. Is the home environment quiet and unhurried or are there numerous activities taking place? Does the family have time to be together as a family unit? This will call for some subtle questions.

6. You should pay close attention to the relationships between the child and his family. Are these close relationships? How does the child get along with his siblings? This will call for both questions and observations.

7. With children in this age group it is extremely important to inquire about the willingness of the parents to work with you on a home program for their child [66]. Your therapy with the preschool-aged child will be almost totally dependent on the parent's home program. Carefully explain what you expect the parents to do, why they would be doing it, how often they should do it, and how long each home session might last. Do not be surprised if the parents agree to work with you but then fail to follow through. At this time you are only interested in the parents' initial response to your request for assistance. The follow through, or lack thereof, will be dealt with later in your therapy.

GETTING THE NEW BEHAVIOR TO OCCUR

GENERAL CONSIDERATIONS

Goal

The goal of this step in therapy is to create easy talking in the clinical environment. With easy talking the client may still have dysfluencies, slight repetitions and/or prolongations, but there will be no emotional involvement and no struggle behaviors. With easy talking the speech rate will be reduced, there will be less effort involved in the speech production, and the speech will flow without inappropriate breaks.

It is at this point that the client should first begin to realize that he can speak normally. This is the beginning of changing the cognitive set.

Speech Objective

Easy talking. Easy talking is a combination of slower rate of speech, careful enunciation, and good speech flow [43]. It is a relaxed, slow, normal speech with careful enunciation and not accompanied by extraneous body movements.

Group and/or Individual Therapy [81–83]

It will be more efficient to teach the easy talking in individual therapy, particularly with young clients. It can be accomplished in a shaping group but it will probably take more time. If this is done in a shaping group you should do it by working individually with the client in a group setting. One advantage of teaching the easy talking in a group setting is the strength of the rewards the client receives from a peer group [86].

The Clinical Stimulus Roles [27-29]

The clinician. During this phase of therapy we want to establish two stimulus roles in the clinical environment. By rewarding the new speech behavior (easy talking) we become associated with the rewards and assume the role of S+. This role then assists in therapy by cuing the new speech behavior to occur when we are present. As the new behavior becomes more predictable and occurs more often, we may, with certain older clients, begin to penalize the occurrences of the old behavior, hard talking. Through this association, we become an S- , cuing these clients not to do hard talking since it will result in penalty.

Other clients. If the therapy is being performed in a shaping group, the members of the group will assume the same S+ role as the clinician as they administer rewards for easy talking. No penalties for hard talking would be used in the group.

Parents. Prior to the client's coming in for therapy the parents have established stimulus roles. If they rewarded the stuttering by being solicitous or overly attentive, their S+ role maintained the stuttering. If they penalized the client for stuttering they maintained the stuttering through the heightened fear and anxiety their S- roles create. To start an effective therapy program we must shift their stimulus roles to an S0, neutralizing their effect on the client [29].

THERAPY PROCEDURES

An Overview

The therapy interaction in this phase of therapy is based on the CIM [23-26] and is directed at teaching the client to do easy talking.

The process that will be used in therapy is that of shaping. The new speech behavior, easy talking, will have to be taught over time, shaping the client's speech behavior closer and closer to easy talking by rewarding more successful performances [31]. The most convenient way to reward the client would be to work in a token economy [31]. This applies to either individual or group therapy.

The easy talking will be taught using modeling, guidance, and information. You will provide the modeling, guidance, and information for the client, even in a group setting [19]. However, as the new speech behavior begins to occur, rewards can be given either by your or by the members of the group [20, 85]. It is the production of the easy talking that is rewarded, not the resultant fluency [43]. The fluency is only a by-product of the use of the easy talking.

The therapy interaction initially will consist of providing modeling, guidance, and information but, as the client becomes more familiar with the new behavior, the interaction changes from a teaching mode to a practice mode and the assistance you provide is faded [20]. In that the client must practice the new behavior, the interaction will be more conversational in nature. The topic of the conversation should be carefully controlled in terms of communication stress [41]. Manipulation of topics to increase communication stress will be used in the next phase of therapy to test the stability of the easy talking.

Therapy Steps

A. Start therapy by placing the child in as comfortable a position as possible. Through a story or by talking in a relaxed manner with the client, get him as relaxed as possible. You should be modeling a relaxed manner and might even provide the client with physical guidance to assist him to relax.

B. As you are achieving relaxation with the client you should be modeling easy talking. You should also be explaining to the client how you are easy talking, that is, speaking slowly, talking relaxed, talking with your lips, and so forth.

C. Ask the client neutral questions as you are achieving relaxation. Evaluate the responses and when the responses show some change toward easy talking, reward the client. Continue to shape the speech until the client can do easy talking in the comfortable, relaxed position. You should introduce gestural cues at this point that are associated with easy talking, such as a hand gesture associated with slower speech and a gesture related to talking with the lips (enunciation).

D. When the client is able to produce easy talking 90% of the time in this clinical environment, move to the next phase of therapy.

Teaching the New Behaviors

The Clinician's Stimulus [19].   *Modeling.* Start by demonstrating the new speech behavior and having the client imitate you. You will probably have to exaggerate the easy talking for the client initially but, as he learns to imitate the model, you can make your model more natural. For example, you might start with counting or short phrases and then work your way up to longer, more natural phrases. Do not be alarmed if the client speaks very softly when he is first using easy talking. As he becomes more comfortable with it, the normal loudness will return.

Should this be occurring in a shaping group where another group member has achieved easy talking, you can use this group member to model the new behavior for the client.

Guidance. There are several forms of guidance you will use with this client. As he attempts to imitate your speech model you can give him gestural guidance in the form of gestures to prompt slower speech and another for more enunciation. These prompts should be used only if the client cannot imitate the easy talking model. Physical guidance can be used to assist the client in relaxation. This might include such things as gently holding the hands to prevent arm movements or holding the knees to eliminate leg movements. This guidance would supplement the verbal guidance you would also be giving the client.

Information. You can give the client behavioral information during his attempts to imitate your speech model. Initially, you should describe what easy talking would sound like and how to do it. You would carefully describe the speech in terms of its being slow and easy and talking with the lips. The amount of information given depends on how soon the client is able to imitate the model, with more information given if the client is having difficulty with imitation.

Stimulus manipulation [29-31]. There are many stimuli in the client's environment that might interfere with his ability to perform the easy talking. You can exert some control over these stimuli to assist the client. To get the client more relaxed, you might want to find a comfortable chair for him. Also, if you are working with the client in a group, you may find that he is unable to perform the new speech behavior in front of the other group members; there are too many stimuli, too much pressure [41]. You will probably have to work with this client outside the group in order to get the new behavior to occur. The topic you choose to talk about is also a matter of concern. If the topic is too sensitive he may not be able to produce the new speech. Choose a neutral or pleasant topic to discuss as he attempts to imitate your speech model.

As the easy talking begins to occur, point out to the client that he is talking a new way and not doing hard talking. This is the first step in changing his cognitive set [49, 56-65].

The client's cognition. [16] As the client perceives your stimulus, he must cogate, or think about it, and then attempt to produce easy talking. If he cannot understand what you want him to do, your stimulus is not appropriate; it is perhaps beyond his ability to comprehend. You must adjust your stimulus to the cognitive level of the client so that he is able to understand what you are presenting to him. His ability to produce the easy talking is directly related to his ability to perceive and comprehend your stimulus.

The client's response [16]. When the client responds he will be attempting to produce easy talking as he perceived it. He will monitor his response but will compare it with his perception of your stimulus.

Note. You can assist the client in performing the easy talking by providing him with gestural guidance, the cues which indicate slower speech and more enunciation.

The clinician's cognitions [20]. The response of the client is the stimulus you will respond to. As the client responds you will make four decisions about the response. You will make decisions about the correctness, frequency, attention, and direction of the next transaction.

1. You will make decisions about the correctness of the response. This is an indication of whether or not the client is learning the new behavior and should be rewarded. The easy talking should improve with successive trials.

2. The frequency of occurrence of the response. If you are using an appropriate reward for the production of the easy talking, it should occur more often. This is your test of the reward you are using.

3. The client's attention to therapy. If the client is motivated, he will be attending to therapy. This is of particular importance with very young children in this age group. The rewards and penalties you use will have a great influence on the attending behaviors of the client. If your rewards and penalties are not appropriate, the client may lose motivation for therapy and not attend to what you are doing. If this is the case, you will have to change your rewards and/or your penalties.

4. How you will start the next transaction. If the client is learning and the easy talking is continuing to improve, you may proceed with your therapy in the next transaction. However, if the speech behavior is incorrect, you will have to repeat the transaction, changing your stimulus. It may be that the client needs a better model, more guidance, or additional information. Your next transaction depends on the results of your testing of the current transaction.

The clinician's response [20–23]. There are three possible responses you can give to your client: a reward, a penalty, or no response at all. It is very important that you respond to the client, and the responses you give to your client during this phase of therapy should be rewards. This creates approach motivation (and attending behaviors) in the client. The rewards presented during this learning period should be on a continuous schedule.

Penalty should be introduced only with certain older clients. These would be clients who are able to produce easy talking but are careless about their use of it. In this event you could introduce a "response cost" penalty, the removal of a token when the hard talking occurs. Because of the ages of these clients, penalty should be used with caution. However, it can be used with some clients to create avoidance motivation to supplement their approach motivation [22].

Rewards [20–22]. Since behaviors that are rewarded occur more often, and you want to encourage the client to use his new easy talking, reward him each time he uses it. However, be careful in selecting a reward. A contingent event is only rewarding if the behavior being rewarded increases in frequency of occurrence. You must decide, before you start therapy, what to use for a reward. You might ask the client what he thinks would be a reward for him or, in a shaping group, what the group might find rewarding. Discuss this with the clients and make them a part of the decision-making process. A response by you or group members is rewarding only if the clients see it in that light.

If you use the token economy, you will be rewarding the client twice, once with the token when the easy talking occurs and again at the end of therapy when he uses his tokens to "purchase" a backup reward [31]. This type of reward system is strongly recommended for clients in this age group. It is also a desirable system to use if there is a home program where the parents will be involved in rewarding the client.

Schedules of rewards [21]. You will use a continuous reward schedule in this phase of therapy. In order to achieve rapid learning of the new speech behavior, this is the best schedule to use.

Penalties [22]. If a client persists in performing hard talking along with easy talking, you might give him some form of feedback, indicating that the hard talking was not correct. Then apply a penalty such as asking him to repeat what he said while using easy talking. However, you must be certain that he can perform easy talking before you penalize the occurrence of hard talking. The penalty used does not have to be harsh. For example, you might say to the client, "You just did hard talking but I know you can use easy talking. Say it again, but this time use easy talking." The reward is encouraging the easy talking and the penalty is discouraging the hard talking.

Changes in Cognitive Set

Clients in this age group usually do not have firmly established negative cognitive sets about their stuttering and themselves. Their cognitive set should be dealt with indirectly. In this stage of therapy the client must learn that he is able to change his stuttering for the better.

If he has had previous therapy and failed, he may have a negative set toward trying therapy again. The best way you can deal with the client's negative set is through success and rewards. However, it is important that you emphasize with the client that *he* is changing the hard talking to easy talking. Point out carefully that you are only teaching him what to do but that he is the one actually doing it. Dwell on this successes, no matter how small they may be. Praise his attempts to change the stuttering through easy talking. Your reward system is extremely important in changing the client's cognitive set.

You may want to deal directly with the cognitive set of some of the older clients in this age group. In this event, use the techniques of having the stutterer create a list of assets [60] and explaining the listener's reaction to hard talking [58].

Home Program

Although the home program will become more important as therapy progresses, the home program for this phase of therapy consists of removing those factors in the home which might be maintaining the stuttering. The most obvious factors would be the parents' rewarding or penalizing their child's stuttering. In so doing, they are working against you as you attempt to create easy talking in therapy.

Remove rewards for stuttering. If the parents are in some way rewarding the child for stuttering, you must remove the reward if you are going to be able to establish easy talking. You should instruct the parents to not react to the stuttering in the home and, if they do this, you can change their stimulus role from an S+ for the old behaviors to an S0 [29]. To accomplish this you will have to work on the parents' cognitive sets [65, 69].

Remove penalty for stuttering. Some parents may be penalizing the child for stuttering in the home. This penalty is creating many negative attitudes in the child and interfering with your attempt to create easy talking. The parents need to be instructed that the penalty is only making the stuttering worse and they should try to ignore the stuttering in the home at this point in therapy. If they will do this you can change their stimulus role from an S- to an S0 for the old behaviors [29]. You will also have to change the cognitive sets of these parents [65, 69].

Monitoring the home program. You must monitor the home program very carefully by creating some sort of a reporting system. The parents must keep you informed as to what is happening in the home. This communication could be in the form of conferences, telephone calls, or written reports depending on the time you have available. The parents are emotionally involved with their child [65, 69] and, not being trained clinicians, they will need a great deal of supervision with the home program.

Working with Teachers

If you can get the cooperation of the client's teacher, you want to deal with her much as you did with his parents. You want to eliminate, as much as possible, any actions by the teacher that might reward or penalize the child's stuttering. Therefore, you should provide her with some information about stuttering in order to change her attitude toward the child and his stuttering, and it is hoped, modify her behavior. An information sheet for teachers is included in Appendix E. This form can be changed according to your own unique situation and sent to teachers whose actions might be interfering with your therapy. It is important to get this information to the client's teacher early in therapy since you may call for her assistance in later phases of therapy.

STABILIZING THE NEW BEHAVIOR

GENERAL CONSIDERATIONS

Goals

The goals here are (1) to stabilize the easy talking so that it occurs in therapy without cues, prompts, or rewards, and (2) to train the client to monitor speech, recognizing hard talking in others and in himself.

In terms of the client's cognitive set, he will now begin to realize that he can use easy talking in the place of hard talking, regardless of the topic, in the clinical environment.

Speech Objectives

(a) During this phase of therapy you want the client to be able to use his easy talking [43] consistently without your assistance, either from prompts or from rewards. There should be at least a 90% reduction in the number of stuttering blocks that he normally has. If dysfluencies still occur, they should resemble normal dysfluencies with no struggle response or emotional involvement. Hard talking should appear in the clinical environment only when the client is under communication stress [41] and only in the early stages of this phase of therapy.

(b) The second objective is to train the client in self-monitoring. Start this by having the client monitor the speech of others. As the monitoring skills are acquired, the client should begin to monitor his own speech, recognizing when hard talking is occurring and shifting to easy talking.

Group and/or Individual Therapy [81–83]

Group therapy has many advantages in this phase of therapy. Not only does it give the client an opportunity to use his new speech behavior in a social situation, it also provides him with an opportunity to interact verbally with other children and to enter discussions of various topics. He learns that he can speak to peers without stuttering and this influences his cognitive set. The group offers another advantage in terms of the second goal of this phase of therapy. Because you want the client to be able to recognize hard talking in others, the other group members could imitate hard talking from time to time to see if the client can catch them. The most serious disadvantage of group therapy is the lack of maturity of the children in this age group. The very young children may not have the maturity to work in a group so individual therapy may be the only approach you can use. Stabilization will occur more rapidly in this setting since there are fewer people involved and you have more control over the clinical environment. In this situation, you will have to serve as the model of hard talking for the client.

The Clinical Stimulus Roles [27–29]

The clinician. The stimulus roles established in the first phase of therapy are now to be altered. The role of S+ shifts from rewards for easy talking which are gradually removed to rewards for catching others doing hard talking. You are now rewarding his recognition of the undesired behavior. When he reaches the point where he recognizes that he is doing hard talking and changes to easy talking, this behavior is given a strong reward. Your role as an S− for the hard talking should gradually fade. Not only should the hard talking appear less often; when it does occur it will not be in its original form. It will be in a very mild form, more likely slightly "sloppy" normal speech.

Other clients. The other members of the shaping group assumed the same roles as the clinician in the first phase of therapy. They will also shift their S+ roles to rewarding the client for catching them doing hard talking or for catching himself talking hard and changing to easy talking. The S− role for hard talking is not used in the group.

Parents. It is now time to actively involve the parents in the therapy program. As you begin to stabilize the easy talking in the clinical environment, you want the parents to begin a home program. They will be working on the client's monitoring skills, his recognition of hard talking when they do it. Their rewards for this recognition will make them an S+, prompting the client to listen for and identify hard talking when he hears it. In that easy talking is being rewarded in therapy, it may occur when the client tells the parents that he has caught them doing hard talking. When this occurs, the parents are to reward him twice, once for monitoring skills and once for using easy talking. The parents are then an S+ for monitoring and an S+ for easy talking.

THERAPY PROCEDURES

An Overview

The CIM continues to be the basis of clinical interaction in this phase of therapy [23–26]. You are not involved in teaching easy talking in this phase of therapy; rather, you are providing the client with an environment where he can practice using easy talking while speaking on a variety of topics and, if in a group situation, interacting verbally with a group of peers. As you move into this phase of therapy, the performance of the easy talking is dependent on the rewards the client receives in therapy. However, you now begin to slowly remove the rewards for easy talking and begin to reward the client for monitoring the speech of others, noting hard talking when it occurs. The rewards for easy talking are shifted to an intermittent schedule while there are continuous rewards for monitoring [21].

The shaping process [31] is still being used. You are now shaping the easy talking to occur in different conversational modes and while speaking about different topics. The emotional content of the topics is gradually increased as the easy talking becomes more stable [41]. You are also shaping the new monitoring skills of the client. Ideally, you are shaping the easy talking in therapy while the parents are shaping the monitoring skills in a home program. However, this can all be done in the therapy environment by shifting the clinical focus from one behavior to another during therapy.

Care must be taken not to move too rapidly in therapy. If the rewards for easy talking are removed too rapidly, the easy talking may slip. In this case, increase the rewards until the easy talking is back to where it was and then remove the rewards more gradually.

The new monitoring behavior should be maintained with continuous rewards. As the monitoring generalizes, the client will begin to monitor his own speech, recognizing when he is doing hard talking. When he recognizes his hard talking and substitutes easy talking, this becomes the behavior that is rewarded. Reward him each time he corrects his own speech.

Therapy Steps

A. The reward schedule for the easy talking is shifted from a continuous reward to an intermittent schedule as the new speech behavior is stabilized. At the same time, the speech monitoring behavior is introduced by having the client indicate when he hears you, a group member, or a parent doing hard talking. The monitoring behavior is continuously rewarded so that it will be learned quickly.

B. Monitor the client's speech carefully to determine the effect of the removal of the rewards. If the speech deteriorates it means that the easy talking is still dependent on a certain amount of reward. To get the easy talking back to the appropriate level, increase your rewards. Once the easy talking is stabilized, you can start fading the rewards again.

C. Your transactions with the client are now mainly in a conversation mode. You are prompting speech through questions, requests for information, or other such stimuli. You are providing the client with an opportunity to practice his new speech behaviors in a social context, in a conversational mode. Your transactional testing now focuses on the stability of the easy talking and occasional testing of the client's monitoring ability as rewards are slowly withdrawn.

D. All transactions are still dependent on the results of the preceding one. If the degree of easy talking continues to be maintained as the rewards are removed, you can continue to remove rewards. If the speech proficiency drops, reevaluate your reward and your reward schedule.

E. As the monitoring skills increase and generalize, the client will begin to notice when he is doing hard talking and will shift to easy talking. This response is heavily rewarded since the client has now achieved a major goal. At this time the models of hard speech by you, group members, or the parents are faded. Rewards are now given to the client for monitoring and changing his speech.

F. When easy talking is occurring 90% of the time, or the client is catching his hard talking and shifting to easy talking, and the rewards have been removed, move to the next phase of therapy.

Stabilizing the New Behavior

The clinician's stimulus [19]. Your clinical focus now is to give the client an opportunity to practice this easy talking while speaking about a variety of subjects. Your stimulus will then be framed in such a way as to elicit as much speech as possible from the client. Avoid asking questions that can be answered in one or two words. Ask the client to tell you about something or describe something. You might ask him to tell you about a vacation, to describe a movie or television program he has seen, or tell you about his hobby. Keep the topics of conversation rather neutral early in this therapy phase. As the easy talking becomes more stable and you are able to remove some rewards, increase the complexity of the topics. You can also introduce more emotional issues such as having him tell you about something he did that was exciting. Remember, communication stress includes both positive and negative emotional responses [41]. You are applying communication stress to the client to see how well he can manage his easy talking under these conditions.

You are also training the client to monitor speech. So, some of your therapy will be directed at teaching the new monitoring behavior. You will first of all identify what the client should be looking for. You will provide the client with a model of hard talking and give him information about what hard talking is. You use words such as "pushing," "struggling," "wiggling," "rushing," and "tense" to describe hard talking. As therapy progresses you will model hard talking during your conversations to see if he can detect it.

The client's cognition [16]. In that you are now requiring the client to converse on various topics, he is going to be attending more to *what* he is saying than *how* he is saying it. He will still be thinking about the rewards for easy talking but not to the degree he was in the previous step of therapy. Further, as therapy progresses and there are fewer rewards, there will be less attending to the performance of the easy talking.

The client is also monitoring your speech. He is looking for signs of hard talking so he can get rewarded for telling you that you are doing hard talking.

The client's response [16]. The client's response is now conversational. He is thinking primarily of what he is talking about. Easy talking should occur consistently. However, hard talking might occur early in this phase of therapy if the topic creates communication stress. If you do hard talking as you talk to the client and he notices it, his response will be to tell you that you were doing hard talking. Also, as a client begins to monitor his own speech, he may interrupt the hard talking and replace it with easy talking.

The clinician's cognitions [20]. Your stimulus is the client's response, his conversational speech, or his monitoring. The decisions you will make are more complicated now since you are judging not only the easy talking, but also the client's monitoring skills. You will make the following decisions about the correctness, frequency, attention, and directions of the transactions.

1. The corrections of the responses. Easy talking: Is the client performing easy talking correctly? If not, you may have moved into this phase of therapy too soon. If the easy talking is correct, you will have to keep some sort of count or record of your rewards so they can be gradually removed.

Speech monitoring: is the client able to differentiate between easy and hard talking? If not, you may have to provide him with a more complete model and more information. If he is making the correct identification, each detection should be rewarded.

2. The frequency of occurrence of the response. Easy talking: The easy talking should be occurring consistently. If it is not, you may need to use a penalty for the hard talking or increase your reward schedule.

Speech monitoring: is the client catching all occurrences of hard talking or is he inconsistent? If he is inconsistent, check the reward to see if it is truly rewarding to the client.

3. The client's attention to therapy. This is an important factor with the younger children in this age group. Your reward is vital here in maintaining motivation and attending behaviors. Although you are not rewarding easy talking as often, you are rewarding the monitoring behaviors. You should be able to maintain the client's attention with this type of reward system.

If the client is not attending to therapy, you can focus your therapy on this factor by penalizing nonattending behaviors and/or rewarding attending behaviors. This reward and penalty system will not disrupt your stabilization program for the easy talking and monitoring.

4. How to initiate the next transaction. While you are in this phase of therapy you will continue to provide the client with an opportunity to use the easy talking in a conversational mode. However, as the behaviors become more stable and independent of the rewards, you should increase the communication stress that the client is experiencing so that he can learn to cope with more stressful talking situations.

You will also be concerned with testing the monitoring skills of the client by doing some hard talking. How you start the next transaction depends on what you are focusing on in therapy at any given time. If you are concentrating on monitoring skills, you may initiate several transactions with hard talking in order to give the client an opportunity to practice the skills and allow you to evaluate his ability.

The clinician's response [20-23]. You will be using the continuous and the intermittent schedules in this phase of therapy, continuously rewarding the monitoring behavior while withdrawing the rewards for easy talking, using an intermittent schedule.

Penalty for hard talking should no longer occur since the client is either using easy talking consistently or, through his monitoring, changing it to easy talking. If the client is not catching all hard talking models, you might use penalty to increase avoidance motivation to speed up the learning of this skill.

Rewards [20-22]. The rewards that you use with clients in this age group are very important. They will be your only means of motivating some of the clients. You must continue to evaluate the effectiveness of your reward to make sure it is still functioning as a reward.

The token economy is strongly recommended as a system to use with clients in this age group. It will solve many of your problems with attempting to find something rewarding for a client, or clients if you are working in a group, and will help you maintain motivation.

If the client is receiving therapy in a group, carefully identify what behavior the client is performing for rewards. In that you are working on two behaviors, easy talking and speech monitoring, it would be best to work on only one at a time in the group.

Schedules of rewards [21]. You will now shift to an intermittent reward schedule for the easy talking, fading all rewards by the end of this phase of therapy. As you introduce the speech monitoring behavior you will use a continuous reward schedule.

Penalty [22]. Penalty should not be used with the group due to the ages of the members and because you are working on two behaviors rather than only one, which complicates the group interaction. Your use of penalty will be primarily for the speech monitoring behavior or the client's nonattending behaviors. If you find that you are consistently having to penalize the client for using hard talking, either the client has lost motivation for therapy or you moved too fast in therapy. If you find yourself in this situation, first reevaluate your penalty. It might be that the client no longer finds the consequence penalizing and has no reason to avoid it. He has then lost his avoidance motivation. The second possibility is that you moved through therapy too rapidly and the client is still having problems producing easy talking. Your penalty is now inappropriate since he cannot produce the easy talking well enough to avoid the penalty. Take this client back a few steps in therapy.

Changes in Cognitive Set

The changes in cognitive set in this phase of therapy concern the client's ability to use easy talking in the clinical environment. He now learns that he can talk on any subject without using hard talking, and if the hard talking does happen, he can change his speech to easy talking. He now has control over his speech in this environment. If the easy talking is occurring at home and his parents are rewarding him for it, he is also beginning to realize that he can use easy talking outside the therapy room. It is still important that the client realize that he is the one who is creating the easy talking.

During this time the stutterer's self-confidence should increase dramatically. There will be changes in his general personality as he becomes less tense, more outgoing, and more verbal. The teachers may report that he is interacting better with his classmates and participating more in classroom activities.

You may want to work directly on changing the cognitive set with older clients in this age group by having them create another list of their assets [60] and going over listener reactions again [58]. These would supplement your general comments and rewards, which are also influencing the cognitive set.

Home Program

The home program now becomes extremely important. You need the parents to help in teaching the client to monitor speech. If you can have them work on the monitoring behavior in the home while you are stabilizing the easy talking in therapy, it makes it easier since the two behaviors are being worked on in two different environments. The home program will be based on a token economy.

Setting up the home program. You begin by preparing the client to play a "game" at home with his parents. Tell him that his parents are going to try and talk hard without his catching them. He will get a token each time he catches them and, after the game is over, he can spend his tokens in his own "store" at home.

Instruct the parents to bring some tokens, such as poker chips, and some small rewards with them to therapy on the day you introduce the home program. Put a price on each reward and then put them away. Now, use the tokens and play a short game with the client, using hard talking on occasions and giving the client a token each time he catches you. The hard talking also serves as a model for the parents since they must be able to do this at home. After a short game where the client wins several tokens, stop the game and count the tokens. Then bring out the rewards and tell the client that he may purchase a reward, pointing out that some rewards only cost one or two tokens but others cost more. The client is then allowed to choose the reward he wants. You might then play another short game and have one of the parents join you. You will have then not only provided the parents with a model of the game, but also involved them in a game so the client associates them with the rewards.

You are now ready to have the parents introduce the game at home. Instruct them to have a game each day, lasting anywhere from 5 to 10 minutes. They should also be instructed to purchase a number of small backup rewards for the "store." It would be best if the parents took the client along when purchasing the rewards so he could choose what he wanted in his store. The rewards are to be kept in a bag or box, out of sight, and not available to the client. When the store is "opened," it should be rather formal with the items laid out on a table and the client allowed to look over the items before he makes a purchase. The purchase is made by taking tokens from the client in payment for an item. Initially the store should be opened every day and then reduced to two or three times a week.

As the game is played, the parents assume an S+ role for speech monitoring through rewarding the behavior. In the event that the client uses easy talking when telling a parent that he or she is doing hard talking, the parents should give him two tokens, one for catching the hard talking and the other for using easy talking. They should make it clear to the client that he is getting tokens for both behaviors. Since the use of penalty must be carefully controlled, it is recommended that it not be used in the home program.

Monitoring the home program. It is important that you know what is happening in the home program, so the parents must keep you carefully informed as to what is transpiring in the game. You need to know how often the client is catching the hard talking, how many tokens he is winning, what he is purchasing, if the parents are keeping the store stocked, and if the client is using easy talking when he catches them. The parents must regularly replace items in the store since the client is selecting the items that are most important to him, the strongest rewards.

The parents can communicate this information to you by telephone or notes if conferences are not possible. Reports should be on a weekly basis unless the parents run into a problem, in which event they should feel free to contact you for advice.

Working With Teachers

If the easy talking is going to occur in the home, it will also appear to some degree in the classroom. You would like to have the occurrences rewarded so the easy talking might appear again. You should attempt to enlist the aid of the client's teacher if at all possible. You will not be asking her to perform time-consuming tasks. Rather, you would ask the teacher to verbally reward the client when he uses his easy talking. You should caution her not to do this in front of the class but to tell the client after class. This is all you would request of the teacher. It would not be appropriate to introduce penalty in this aspect of your therapy program.

If you have not already sent the teacher information on stuttering, do it now. The information sheet in Appendix E can be copied and sent or modified in any way you see fit. With this information, the teacher should be able to provide you with some invaluable assistance.

GENERALIZING THE NEW BEHAVIOR

GENERAL CONSIDERATIONS

Goals

The goal in this phase of therapy is to get the easy talking to occur in talking environments outside the clinic room. We want the client to carry over the new speech into his everyday life and be able to maintain his normal-sounding speech in all speaking situations.

It is at this point of therapy that the client comes to realize that he can control his speech in all talking situations. This is a major change in his cognitive set, the point where he begins to realize and believe that he does not have to go through life being afraid of stuttering.

Speech Objective

The speech objective is essentially the same as in the previous phase of therapy, except that we now want the client to use the easy talking in all talking situations. As the easy talking becomes more stable in other environments, we would again expect it to occur 90% of the time, regardless of where the client is or what he is talking about. His speech is now normal-sounding even though there may be times when the easy talking is characterized by small and effortless dysfluencies, which are typical in the speech of most younger children. If, due to stress, carelessness, or some other factor, his speech approaches hard talking, we would expect the client to recognize it and shift to easy talking.

Group and/or Individual Therapy [81–83]

This phase of therapy lends itself to either group or individual therapy. The client is now using his easy talking in the clinical environment, and if there is a home program, to some extent in the home. The main focus of therapy now is to get reports on how well the client is using his easy talking in all speaking situations. With older clients in this age group we can get this information through reports either to the clinician in individual therapy or to the members of a shaping group. Individual therapy would give the clinician a better opportunity to analyze his reports but the group would be able to provide stronger rewards for motivation to work on the speech outside therapy. This is an important factor since rewards are now being given for work outside rather than on the speech production in the clinical setting. The rewards, particularly from peers, will have a positive influence on his cognitive set. Penalty can also be used in either group or individual therapy. The penalty is not directed toward the speech production (unless needed) but is used to make certain that the client is using the easy talking outside therapy [87]. If he is not using his easy talking outside, penalty from a peer group will have a greater impact than from the clinician in creating avoidance motivation.

Group therapy also offers you an advantage if the client is facing extremely frightening talking situations. If they are so frightening that he cannot use his easy talking in them [28], you can role play them in the group, reducing the fear of the situation to the point where the client can use his new easy talking in it [30].

With the very young client, group therapy may not be an option. In this case, generalization of the easy talking must be accomplished in individual therapy and in the home program.

The Clinical Stimulus Roles [27–29]

We are now at a crucial point in therapy regarding discriminative stimuli. The client is using his new speech behavior, easy talking and speech monitoring, in the clinical environment because there are so many S+ cues. He is "reminded" or prompted to use the new behavior whenever he sees the clinician or any member of the group since they have rewarded the behavior in the past. He may also be using the behavior in the home if the parents have become S+ through rewarding it. We must attempt to create as many new S+ outside the clinic room as possible so that the behavior is prompted when the client is in a variety of environments. We can accomplish some of this by shifting S-situations to S+ so they will prompt the new behavior rather than the old one.

The clinician. We will continue our S0 role for the client's speech as we fade the rewards for his monitoring. However, in that he will be making reports to us in one form or another on his work outside, we will assume an S+ role for the work outside therapy. We will reward him for his use of easy talking and self-monitoring in outside talking situations. We will probably even assume an S- role if he is not doing his outside assignments and we have to penalize him for it. With the preschool child we will also be an S+ for use of easy talking and monitoring but we are dependent on the parent's reports on how often the behaviors are occurring and how correct they are when they happen.

Other clients. If the client is working in a shaping group, the other members have assumed the role of an S0 for the easy talking and speech monitoring. If the client reports on his outside activities to the other group members, they will assume the same roles as the clinician: an S + for the outside work and an S- if the client is not doing all of his assignments.

Parents. The parents have become S+ for both speech monitoring and easy talking. We are now going to focus on their role as an S+ for easy talking by making changes in the home program. Their S+ role is extremely important as we introduce the easy talking into environments such as restaurants, stores, friends' homes, and so forth.

Other people and objects. The more S+ you can create, the easier it will be for the client to use the new speech behavior outside. You already have the other members of the group who function as an S+ whenever the client sees them in school. If you can get a teacher to reward him when he uses the new behavior (privately, of course), over a short period of time that teacher will also become an S+. You could even have the client bring in a close friend who could give the client rewards. This is a good S+ but be careful, since if their friendship ends, there could be some problems. We can also have objects as an S+ such as the record book.

The Record Book [60–64]

The record book serves the same functions as does the log book, differing only in terms of who keeps the records and how complete they are. In that children in this age group have little or no writing skills, the record keeping is modified so that either the parent can keep the records or the older child can use symbols to record his use of easy talking. The record book is very important in this phase of therapy since it is our only source of information concerning the client's use of easy talking outside the clinical environment. You will have to adjust the record book to each individual client according to writing skills, cognitive level, and maturity. Perhaps the most difficult task you will have will be to establish some means of determining the level of communicative stress in each speaking situation [61].

THERAPY PROCEDURES

An Overview

The easy talking is now occurring but not where needed, in talking situations outside therapy. You must transfer it to other talking environments. We are now shifting the focus of our therapy to the antecedent events, that is, the various S+ and S- in the client's life, and will manipulate these so that new S+ encourage the easy talking to occur, including shifting S- talking situations to either an S0 or an S+. You will be concentrating on stimulus control in this phase of therapy [27–31].

An important aspect of therapy now is to develop some way the client can record his success in using the easy talking in other talking situations. To record these attempts we will use the record book [60–64]. With older clients you can make specific assignments as to the number of practices you want each day. Instruct the client to start his practice in less stressful situations in order to increase the probability of success. With the very young clients you will have to depend on the parents to record the client's use of easy talking and you will not be able to structure the client's practices as you can with the older clients.

You are now asking the client to give reports, written and/or oral, on how well he is able to use his easy talking outside the clinic room. Your stimulus to the client is usually in the form of asking for information. If the client has had a problem with a particular talking situation, you may rehearse it with him so he has a better chance to use his easy talking the next time he is in that situation. With younger children you will depend on the record book from the parents to determine how well the client is using his easy talking outside therapy. Regardless of the form of the report, verbal and/or the record book, the client is given many rewards for his outside work and his success in using his new behaviors.

You are still shaping the easy talking but you are now concerned about its occurrence in situations with differing amounts of communication stress. With the older clients in this age group you might be able to explain to the client that he will have better speech in less stressful situations than in more difficult ones [41, 61].

Therapy Steps

A.   As you move into this phase of therapy you are no longer rewarding the easy talking in therapy. You now have to introduce the client to the idea of practicing his easy talking outside of therapy. You explain that, like riding a bicycle, you have to practice to learn how to do something new. You will also have to explain how he is to practice. He should be told that he practices when he makes a special effort to do easy talking. Therapy will now consist of evaluating the client's speech efforts outside of therapy. With the very young client you will have to explain to the parents how they are to keep the record book and why you need it.

B.   After you have introduced the concept of the record book to the client, check it carefully during the next few therapy sessions to make sure the client understands what you want him to do. You may have to explain the record book carefully several times before he comprehends it. Even if the reports in the record book are incorrect at first, reward the client for his effort to use his easy talking. It is these rewards that will make the record book an S+ for the client.

You will also have to review the parents' record book with them to make sure they are recording the client's use of easy talking. They will need very specific instructions on what information to record.

C.   When the record book from either a client or a client's parents is being filled out correctly, go over the book carefully with the client [64]. Find something positive in each report so you can reward his effort. Point out how many good reports there are and how well he is using easy talking. Reward his willingness to use his easy talking. With the older client it is very important that he understands that the stress in speaking situations will influence the quality of his easy talking.

D.   The clinical transactions are now focusing on the client's cognitive set. You are emphasizing his successes with his easy talking. If there is a talking situation where the older client feels he failed (the easy talking did not occur) you can still reward him for his effort.

E. As you proceed in this phase of therapy, have the older client use his easy talking in more difficult situations [41, 61]. He may have limited his practices to talking to his friends and his family. Have him work up to practicing in more difficult situations such as answering a question in class. Move slowly so that the practices are successful.

Generalizing the New Behavior

The clinician's stimulus [19]. Your stimulus now is most often in the form of questions about the client's practicing of his new behavior outside therapy. You will ask him about a report from his record book. Have him tell you how successful he was in using his easy talking. Discuss the most successful situations with him in some detail. You will also be asking him if the easy talking is occurring when he is not specifically practicing. The easy talking should begin to occur spontaneously and these occurrences should also be rewarded. With the younger client, you will be getting the information on the occurrence of easy talking from the record book the parents are keeping.

The client's cognitions [16]. The most important part of your therapy now is the client's cognitions about his speech. You are providing evidence through the record book that he can successfully use his easy talking outside therapy. His cognitive set has been changed somewhat in previous phases of therapy but it is at this point where he learns that he can control his speech in all talking situations. It is here that the client learns to trust his ability to control his speech. This is where his confidence is built up, his new self-concept is formed, his fears decrease, and so forth. You are now working more with the stutterer than the stuttering.

The client's response [16]. The client is now responding to your questions about his use of easy talking outside therapy. As he is telling you about the experiences in the record book, you will be hearing a reflection of his cognitive set. If he focuses on the negative parts of the reports, this is a manifestation of his negative set. You should counter this with a positive review of the report.

The clinician's cognitions [20]. You will be attending more to what the client is telling you than to how well he is using his easy talking during the report. If the client is using hard talking in his reporting, you might remind him to monitor his speech and use easy talking or you could use the cues you introduced in the preceding phase of therapy. Should hard talking occur repeatedly, you should carefully consider if this client should be in this phase of therapy. During the client's report you will be evaluating the following:

1. The correctness of the response. You are most interested in how well the client was able to use his easy talking and, with the older client, if he did all of the assignments. There are two sources of information for you. First, you are interested in the reporting in the record book. Have the client tell you about more successful talking experiences and how he interprets them. The second source of information is the home program. Check with the client and see how he feels he is doing. If he is having great success you will want to reward him for doing so well at home. However, if the client is not succeeding, you should reevaluate the home program and make changes to increase the client's success.

2. The frequency of occurrence of the response. The record book and/or the home program will give you an indication of how often the easy talking is occurring outside therapy. If easy talking is not occurring more often, the rewards the client is receiving may have lost their effectiveness or the schedule of receiving them is not adequate and you will have to modify your therapy and/or the home program.

3. The client's attention to therapy. Even though therapy now consists of evaluating the record book and/or the home program, you will still be providing the client with rewards. This should maintain the client's motivation and attention. This will be more difficult with the younger client but as long as you have an appropriate reward that the client wants to achieve, you will be able to maintain his attention. The token economy will prove extremely valuable here since the backup rewards are always appropriate.

4. How to initiate the next transaction. If the client has not fully comprehended his success in a practice, you may want to take the next transaction to emphasize how well he did. This also applies to a report on how well the client has done in the home program. You want to emphasize the client's successes and the following transaction, or transactions, can be focused on pointing out how well the client did. Once you feel that the client understands and appreciates his success, you can move on to the next report.

The clinician's response [20–23]. You are now rewarding the client's use of easy talking outside therapy. With younger clients you will be dependent on the parent's record book and the report on the home program. The older client may be able to keep his own record book and this will allow you to provide more rewards, since the client is involved not only in doing his assignments, but also in directly practicing his easy talking.

Penalty can be used in two ways. First, it can be used with older clients who do not do all of their assignments for their record book. Second, it can be used with clients who persist in using both hard and easy talking. To discourage the use of hard talking, you can penalize its occurrence. However, this should be done with caution, particularly with the very young client.

Rewards [20–22]. The rewards the client receives from you and, perhaps, his parents, will supplement those he is receiving from his easy talking. With younger clients you should use tangible rewards such as stickers or stamps in their record book, paired with verbal praise to strengthen the reward. You should also have a means of rewarding their reports of their success in the home program and their use of easy talking in general speech. This is where tokens are convenient. The main problem you face in generalizing the new speech behavior is that your rewards are not contingent upon the easy talking. Your work with the client's record book will enable him to associate the reward with the practices and the successes he has had.

If the client is reporting on his practices in a shaping group, point out the client's successes to the group and have them reward him. Even though you may have to carefully structure this in the group, it does not weaken the reward [86]. The reward from the peer group is very strong and helps to motivate the client as he takes his easy talking out into new environments.

Schedules of rewards [21]. You are now going to have to shift back to a very heavy reward schedule. The client will need as much reward as possible for practicing his speech outside the therapy room and succeeding in the home program.

Penalty [22]. Penalty is now directed toward failure to complete outside assignments or for persistent use of hard talking. If you are penalizing a client for continuing to use hard talking even though he can do easy talking, use the penalty carefully. You do not want to create anxiety or tension in the client since this will increase the occurrence of hard talking. If you are using a token economy you might introduce the penalty in the form of a game. Place a number of tokens on the table and when the client does easy talking give him a token; but if he does hard talking, you take one. In this way, you are not taking the token directly from the client, but he still loses one. You should structure this procedure so that the client recognizes that the penalty is for hard talking. The game should be structured so that the client "wins" every game even though you may get some of the tokens. If the client is reporting to a group of peers, any penalty is strong and you will have to monitor the amount carefully. You do not want to demoralize the client with too much penalty.

Changes in Cognitive Set

At this point in therapy, the client realizes that he can use his easy talking in all speaking situations, and further changes in cognitive set will occur. In going over the record book and the home program you should stress that he is doing easy talking and the hard talking has gone away. Talk with him about how he enjoys using his easy talking.

The client's self-confidence should increase even more in this phase of therapy. He will be using his easy talking in a variety of speaking situations and will no longer be fearful of speaking. His peer relationships will also improve since he is now willing and able to enter into such relationships. General behavior, both in the home and in school, will also improve because the client is less defensive and does not have to compensate by getting peer recognition through attention-getting behaviors in the classroom or in school.

Home Program

You now need to modify the home program to meet the goals of this phase of therapy. The focus of the home game shifts to the client's easy talking as the parents fade out their hard talking. The client is told that he can now get tokens two ways, by catching his parents doing hard talking or by using easy talking when he talks. As the parents' hard talking occurs less frequently, the focus is shifted to the easy talking. The game now consists of the parents conversing with the client about his activities in school, projects he is working on, or having the client tell them a story or tell them about a movie or television program he has seen. The purpose of this is to get the client to talk as much as possible during the 5 or 10 minutes set aside for the game. The schedule of rewards is now shifted to an intermittent schedule.

When the client is able to maintain his easy talking for the entire game period, the program is again modified. The client is now told that not only can he get tokens for easy talking in the game, but if he does any easy talking after the evening meal, he will get a token. The parents are instructed to reward any easy talking which occurs in the evening. Because the client is using easy talking both in therapy and in the game, it may already be occurring to some degree during this time. Whenever easy talking occurs in this new time period, it is continuously rewarded for a brief time for rapid learning and then intermittently to resist extinction when the rewards are faded. It is also at this point that the parents begin to keep the record book of the client's use of easy talking. The record book is reviewed with the client by both the parents and you. The client now receives two rewards for his use of easy talking, one from the parents and the other from you. Remember that penalty is not used in the home program.

The easy talking should begin to occur on a regular basis during the evening and should also begin to occur during all speech in the home since the parents and the home itself are now S+ for the client. The parents are then instructed to reward the occurrences of easy talking at any time and in any environment. If they are shopping and the client asks a question using easy talking, he is given a reward immediately. This is the procedure used to generalize or transfer the easy talking to all of the client's speaking environments.

Monitoring the home program. Communication between you and the parents is vital. You must know how well the client is doing in using his easy talking in the home and in other environments. You also need to know how the parents are responding to the client's record book as they review it with him. In the early stages of this phase of therapy you will be primarily concerned with the easy talking in the home; but, as therapy progresses, your concern will shift to his speech performance in other environments. The information you receive about the client's performance in the home program will prove to be a valuable supplement to the information you have available in his record book. With the younger client, where the parents are keeping a record book, it would be wise to have them send the book with the client each week. You can then review the record book with the client and contact the parents if you have any questions or suggestions.

You have been having the parents act as clinicians for their child in the home program during the last two phases of therapy. It is in this phase that you begin to concentrate on training them to expand their role as clinicians; to begin to plan their own home program, to work out ways of recording their child's speech, and so forth. You should be discussing your therapy with them and allowing them to gain insight into how you deal with any problem that might arise. This training is essential, because you will have to depend on the parents to carry on the maintenance program to follow.

Working With Teachers

By this time in therapy the client should have a number of S+ cuing the easy talking to occur, including you, the record book, other clients in the group, and even your clinic room. You can now expect the easy talking to occur occasionally in the classroom. The client's teacher may become a valuable S+ at this time. She can assume this role by simply rewarding the client when he uses his easy talking. If she is consistent in her rewards, telling him after class how well he did, she will quickly assume this role. You do not want to introduce penalty in this situation.

To enlist the help of the teacher, you will need to have a conference with her and explain exactly what easy talking is and how she should reward the client. If this is the first time you have approached the teacher, you should provide her with the information about stuttering for the teacher in Appendix E. However, if the teacher was involved in the previous step of therapy, you need only ask her to continue rewarding the client and explain the new goals of this phase of therapy.

MAINTAINING THE NEW BEHAVIOR

GENERAL CONSIDERATIONS

With children in the 2- to 8-year-old age group we face some unique problems in the last phase of therapy. Some of the older clients have both the motivation to work on their speech and the cognitive ability to comprehend our therapy, while others have neither the motivation nor the cognitive ability to understand the long-term ramifications of our therapy. The latter are those clients who are in therapy because their parents decided that the child's stuttering was a problem. This section of therapy addresses problems that arise in dealing with clients without motivation or highly developed cognitive skills. For the more mature clients, you are referred to the maintenance phase of therapy for clients aged 9 through adult. With a little planning you will be able to adapt the maintenance program presented there for these clients.

With the younger clients we must determine who will assume the responsibility of maintaining the easy talking and how they will do this. Since our treatment program is heavily dependent on parental involvement, most of the responsibility will rest with the parents. However, in terms of the general maintenance program, you are both directly and indirectly involved. Your direct involvement concerns your continuing to train the parents to be their child's clinician while your indirect involvement is the periodic contact with the client to assess how well he is maintaining his easy talking. Let us first consider the role of the parents.

Parents

Throughout therapy you have been training the parents to be the client's clinician. They have not only been given information about stuttering as you worked on their cognitive set, but also you have worked with them on the therapy program that they carried on in the home.

It is now time to bring this training into focus so they can function as the clinician for their child.

The parents' responsibility consists primarily of monitoring the child's speech in all speaking environments to make sure the easy talking is maintained. They have been gradually removing their rewards for easy talking. If the easy talking has become rewarding in and of itself, it will continue to occur. However, because the client's speech in the home environment will, probably, be all easy talking, the parents may begin to take it for granted that it is occurring at the same level of proficiency in all talking situations. They must check the speech outside the home in a variety of situations, including checking with the client's teacher. In the event that hard talking begins to occur, the parents must reinstate the home program they used in the generalization phase of therapy. Perhaps all the child needs is a brief reminder to use the easy talking. When the easy talking is consistent again, the rewards can be removed at a faster rate than the first time the child went through this routine. The maintenance program may go on for several months so the parents must continue their monitoring of their child's speech until the easy talking occurs consistently in all talking situations over a period of at least 3 months. Even after this goal has been reached, the parents should continue to be aware of the quality of the child's speech.

Clinician

Your task is to work with the parents in maintaining the client's new speech. You will continue training them to act as a clinician by discussing potential problems with them and assisting them in planning ways to deal with the problems. As in the example above, you might ask them what they would do if the hard talking began to reappear. They should be able to review the therapy that they have carried on in the home and decide what phase should be repeated in order to eliminate the hard talking. You should not provide them with the answer, but, rather, lead them to the solution of the problem. If they understand the basic principles involved in the therapy program, they should be able to decide what to do if a problem arises.

In the event that the child is in school, you should arrange to see him periodically to see how well he is maintaining his easy talking. You can also check with his teachers about his speech. If a problem arises, the parents should be the first to deal with it under your guidance. You should not immediately bring the client back into an active therapy program, since this would defeat the parents' role as clinician to their child. Reinstatement in active therapy should occur only as a last resort.

Although it is agreed among professional clinicians that there is no cure for stuttering, there is some question about whether this applies to the very young stutterer, especially the preschool child. Is there a need for a maintenance program which will continue for the rest of the child's life or will the child, after learning easy talking, speak normally from that time on? There is no research to help us here, but in my experience with this therapy program for very young stutterers, I lean toward the belief that easy talking will continue. Because the cognitive set of the very young stutterer has not been severely influenced by the stuttering, the therapy seems to be able to remove not only the hard talking, but also the negative aspects of the cognitive set so the child no longer thinks as a stutterer or thinks of himself as a stutterer. If there is a cure for stuttering, we will probably find it first in the very young stutterer.

Chapter 10

Treatment: Age 9 Through Adult

The treatment program described here is designed for clients from 9 years of age through adulthood. It is based on the cognitive level of the client and his writing ability. In this program we deal with individual speaking behaviors (rate, enunciation, easy onset, and flow—REEF) to achieve control over the stuttering. The client must be able to understand the concept of individual behaviors making up a new way to speak. He must also be able to write down a record of his experiences with his new speech behavior as he uses it outside the clinic room. Some of the younger children in this age group may not have the cognitive or writing skills necessary for this form of treatment. If you feel that a client might have difficulty with these aspects of this program, use the program for younger children, which does not rely on these skills.

FACTORS INFLUENCING THIS THERAPY PROGRAM

Because of the wide age range of clients you will use this program with, there are some important factors which will influence your therapy. Take these into consideration as you adapt the treatment program to the individual client and to your clinical environment.

Client Motivation [71–75]

The motivation for therapy will vary according to the age and maturity of the client. The older client is more likely to recognize the long-term implications of his stuttering and be motivated to work on his speech. The younger client will be emotionally involved in his stuttering but may lack some motivation because of his inability to see the stuttering as a long-term problem in his life. There is also the adolescent who, perhaps because of peer pressure, will have little or no motivation to work on his speech. Motivation is an important part of the effectiveness of your therapy, and you will have to create it for the unmotivated client.

Peer Pressure [50, 74]

The basic need to be accepted by peers influences the cognitive set of the client and this in turn can create problems in terms of your therapy program. He may resist therapy because of the "stigma" of having to be taken out of class for therapy, an indication that there is something "wrong" with him. He may also be resistant in terms of taking his new speech behavior out of the therapy room for fear that his peers may laugh at him. All stutterers are influenced by peer pressure but the adolescent is particularly susceptible.

Parent Influence — Home Program [71–75]

The influence of the parents on the client will vary according to the client's age. With younger children in this age group the parents are still an important factor in the child's life and if it is possible to set up a home program, it will provide a valuable supplement to your therapy. If, with a younger client, you have no opportunity to set up a home program and you feel it is a necessary component of your therapy, you will have to compensate for the lack of support by enlisting the help of significant others in the client's life. With the adolescent, the relationship between the individual client and his parents can vary from a cooperative relationship to rebellion. With older clients the influence of the parents decreases and a home program would depend on the age of the client and the relationships between him and his parents. The effectiveness of a home program decreases with the age of the client.

The Therapy Program

In that you are providing your clinical services in the school environment, there are specific procedures and protocols which are dictated for you through federal regulations, specifically Public Law 94-142. A quick reference guide to these procedures and protocols is provided for you in Appendix D. The implementation of the following treatment program will be influenced by these regulations, and different states and districts have additional rules and regulations. Modify the following treatment program according to your district's regulations.

EVALUATION

THE STUTTERING

Assessment of the Speech

The first step in the evaluation is to determine if the individual is actually stuttering or is only displaying normal dysfluencies [38]. You should focus on the individual's emotional involvement in the speech dysfluencies which will be manifested by noticeable body tension, excessive body movement, secondary mannerisms, struggle behavior, and other behaviors not usually associated with normal speech dysfluencies.

Having determined that the individual is stuttering, evaluate the speech using either a formal or informal stuttering evaluation procedure (severity scales) [34]. This evaluation will give you both an indication of the severity of stuttering and a detailed account of the stuttering behaviors before therapy. This will give you a means of measuring your clinical progress.

Descriptions of Secondary Mannerisms [36–37]

If you use an informal scale, be sure to include information about secondary mannerisms, such as how often the behavior is used, how intense or strong the behavior is when it occurs, and how long the behavior lasts once it occurs. For example, if the client blinks his eyes during a block, your description might be as follows: eye blinks occur immediately after the block starts, four or five blinks occur during the block, they are very intense when they occur, and the eyebrows are involved in the eye blink.

Some forms of secondary mannerisms are very difficult to detect, such as word substitution and circumlocution. You may have to ask the client if he is substituting words. In some instances you can observe him attempt to say one word and substituting another word. Circumlocutions are even more difficult to detect and the client may not be able to report this to you. Evaluate the speech carefully, and if you detect word substitutions and/or circumlocutions, make note of it.

Speech Samples [34, 96]

If possible, you should evaluate the client's speech under three conditions: conversation, reading, and story telling. Conversational speech tests the speech under spontaneous conditions; reading tests the speech where word substitutions are not possible; and story telling tests the speech under conditions of thinking/talking or propositionality.

THE STUTTERER

In addition to the direct evaluation of the stuttering behaviors, you will want to learn about the client's attitudes, emotions, and feelings [55–56]. You need to know how he views his stuttering and himself. Do not assume that if his stuttering appears rather mild to you, the listener, that the client will have a mild reaction to it.

Determine Attitudes About:

The stuttering [50–53]. In order to determine how the client feels about his stuttering, you have to be rather direct in your questions. Some questions you might ask your client are listed below, but you should add questions according to your particular client. Try to avoid asking questions that can be answered in a single word.

Why do you think you stutter?

What do you do when you stutter?

Do you get angry with yourself when you stutter and, if so, why?

How frightening is it when your stuttering happens?

What do other people do when you stutter?

The parents' responses [50, 65–67, 69]. It is important to determine the parents' response to the younger client when he stutters. Ask the client what his parents do when he stutters. You may find that each parent responds differently. This information might give you insight into factors that might be maintaining the stuttering. You may also gain some insight into problems you will have to deal with when you meet the parents at the IEP Conference. You might ask some of the following questions:

What does your mother do when you stutter?

What does your father do when you stutter?

What has your mother or father said to you about your stuttering?

Peer responses [50, 74]. In that the client spends a good share of his time in school with his peers, you should determine how the client feels his peers react when he stutters. This is especially important with older clients in this group, since they are in adolescence and peer pressure is a factor you have to deal with in therapy. You have to expand these questions according to the age and sex of your client.

How do boys (or men) your age react when you stutter?

How do girls (or women) your age react when you stutter?

Do the other students say anything to you when you stutter?

Responses of "others" [50, 53]. Your client will also have opinions about how his listeners, in general, react to his stuttering. His interpretation of listener reaction is an important part of his overall attitude toward his stuttering. You might ask some of the following questions:

What do people think of you when you stutter?

What do people think of your stuttering?

How do people act when you stutter to them?

The client's responses [50–53]. You should determine what the client does when his listener reacts to his stuttering. How does he feel and what does he do when his listener reacts to his stuttering? A few of the questions you might ask are:

What do you do or think when your listener smiles when you stutter?

What do you do or think when your listener frowns when you stutter?

What do you do when someone teases you about your stuttering?

The client's self-concept [49–50]. On a more general level, you need to determine what the client thinks of himself. You need to determine the effect of the stuttering on the client's self-concept. How have his repeated failures to correct his speech affected his self-concept? Expand these questions according to the age and sex of your client. Some questions to ask are:

Tell me all the good things about you.

What is there about you that you do not like?

What do you think of the person you see when you look in a mirror?

Previous therapy [51, 54]. Your client has more than likely had treatment for his stuttering from other clinicians. It is important for you to find out what he thinks about the therapy he has had. If he has a negative attitude toward his previous therapy, you may have to work with his attitude before starting your own therapy. You also need to know what procedures previous clinicians used with the client. You may find yourself repeating procedures other clinicians have used and that the client has negative attitudes toward. You might ask the following questions:

What other therapy have you had for your stuttering?

What kinds of things did you do in therapy?

How much did your therapy help you with your speech?

Are you still able to use some of the things you learned in therapy?

Observations and Judgments to Make

In addition to asking questions, you can learn a great deal about your client by observing him during your evaluation. Some of the more important things for you to observe include the client's verbal level, his assertiveness, and sensitive areas in his life.

Verbal/nonverbal. How verbal is the client? If the client is reacting to his stuttering by withdrawing he will be relatively nonverbal. He will answer questions in the shortest way possible and will rarely volunteer speech. Other clients may be very verbal even though they are quite severe stutterers. This will give you some insight into how the stutterer copes with his stuttering and this attitude will influence your therapy.

Assertive/nonassertive. More typically, you will find that the stutterer is withdrawn and nonassertive. The client may speak softly and be quite nonverbal. He may also rarely look at you when speaking. On the other hand, there are some stutterers who are quite assertive in spite of their stuttering. They are outgoing, speak up, are verbal, and maintain eye contact with you even while they are stuttering. However, beware of making a judgment based solely on eye contact. There are cultures where direct eye contact is interpreted as an act of hostility and individuals influenced by these cultures do not maintain eye contact [53]. The client's assertiveness will have a significant influence on your therapy. Assertive clients will be more willing to use new speech behaviors outside the therapy environment.

Sensitive issues. There are probably sensitive topics or issues for the client which, when discussed, create more stuttering. You should determine these topics or issues in order to avoid them in early therapy and to use them to test his control over this speech later in therapy. Issues you should check into are (a) peer relationships, (b) relationships with the opposite sex, (c) interaction with parents, and (d) school environment.

General adjustment. The overall adjustment of the client should also be considered. You should attempt to determine how the client has adjusted to his environment. You will have to check with the parents and teachers to gather this information. Investigate the following areas:
   (1) relations with peers, male and female
   (2) classroom behavior
      (a) class clown
      (b) behavior problems
      (c) withdrawn
   (3) home environment.

CONFERENCE WITH PARENTS

PRESENT PROBLEM TO PARENTS

When you discuss your findings with the parents in the IEP Conference, it is important to remember that the parents do not understand the complexities of stuttering and, further, are emotionally involved in it with their child [65]. Avoid the use of professional jargon and use terms that the parents understand. One of the most difficult factors you have to present to the parents is the client's emotional reaction to his stuttering [49–54]. You should make sure that the parents have a basic understanding of the problem and how you plan to treat it [95–101]. If the parents agree that their child may receive therapy, you should get as much information from them as possible to assist you with your therapy.

AREAS TO EXPLORE WITH PARENTS

1. You should determine the parents' feelings as to why their child stutters [38, 65]. This may be the source of much anxiety in the home, and of parental negative reactions to the child.

2. Ask the parents how they respond to the child when he stutters. There are only three possible responses: to reward the client by being solicitous, to penalize the client by a negative reaction, or to ignore the stuttering [65]. The last response will be rare since most parents will have some overt response to their child's stuttering.

3. Another important area of questioning concerns the reactions of siblings when the child stutters [50]. Your questions should include both younger and older siblings.

4. Friends are a peer group for the client. Ask the parents how his friends react when he stutters [50].

5. The home environment should be carefully examined. Is the home environment quiet and unhurried or are there numerous activities taking place? Does the family have time to be together as a family unit? This examination calls for some subtle questions.

6. You should pay close attention to the relationships between the client and his family. Are these close relationships? How does the client get along with his siblings? This calls for both questions and observations.

7. It is important to inquire about the willingness of the parents to work with you on a home program for their child [66]. You should carefully explain what you expect them to do, why they would be doing it, how often they should do it, and how long each home session might last. Do not be surprised if the parents agree to work with you but then fail to follow through. At this time you are only interested in the parent's initial response to your request for assistance. The follow through, or lack thereof, will be dealt with later in your therapy.

INFORMATIONAL MEETINGS WITH CLIENT

Informational meetings with the client are used to give him information about stuttering. You need to give him insight into what stuttering is, where it occurs in speech, what precipitates it, the role that stress plays in stuttering, and other factors [33–42, 56–59].

There are two goals in this phase of therapy. First, you want to reduce the general fear of stuttering, and you can accomplish this through the information since the more we understand something the less we fear it. Second, you are starting to effect a change in the client's cognitive set toward his stuttering. Both of these factors will make your therapy more effective and more efficient.

WHAT STUTTERING IS

The concept of stuttering can be explained by comparing it to a two-layer cake. The first layer is repetitions, the second layer is prolongations. All stuttering cakes have both layers.

Repetitions [35, 40]

Explain that repetitions occur when the client is attempting to change mouth positions and the repetitions are the stuttering block. A repetition on a voice consonant such as a (d) can be either voiced or unvoiced. The unvoiced repetition will be heard as a repetition of the (t) sound as in "t-t-t-t-dog." You should demonstrate this for the client.

Prolongations [35, 40]

The client should understand that prolongations can occur on mouth positions or sounds, and that they are another form of the stuttering block. You should demonstrate to the client that he can have a prolongation on a (b) position although there will be no voice or movement. The prolongation on a vowel may be voiced as a prolongation or as an unvoiced mouth position as the stutter holds his breath.

Secondary Mannerisms [36]

The secondary mannerisms should be explained to the client as anything he does to avoid, or get out of, the stuttering block. You should emphasize that, over time, secondary mannerisms lose their effectiveness, no longer avoiding or releasing the block, but they remain as part of the stuttering pattern. The frosting of the stuttering cake is made up of the various secondary mannerisms the stutterer adopts. The "stuttering cake" has many layers of frosting since the stutterer never gives up a secondary mannerism, he just adds new ones.

WHERE STUTTERING OCCURS IN SPEECH [39, 56]

Most stutterers think that they have stuttering blocks on sounds. You should explain that the block occurs on the *transitions* between sounds rather than on the sounds themselves. You can demonstrate this for the client by stuttering in the following three ways on the word "MAN."

1. "Muh-muh-muh-man." You have said the (m) sound four times, but you did not shift the mouth into the correct position for the (a) sound. Point out that there is no (uh) sound in the word "man."

2. "uh-uh-uh-man." The problem here is that you did not shift the mouth into the (m) position to start the word.

3. "mmmmmmmmmman." The problem is quite similar to the repetition. You are prolonging the (m) sound because you did not shift the mouth into the position for the (a) sound.

You should also emphasize that most stuttering occurs when the stutterer begins to speak [40], and that the more he stops to "prepare" for words, the greater his chances of stuttering [45]. The stutterer has problems getting his speech started, but once it is started the likelihood of stuttering is greatly reduced.

SOURCES OF COMMUNICATION STRESS [41]

Stuttering occurs when there is some form of communication stress. If the stutterer is alone in a room or talking to a very young child, there is no stress and there will be no stuttering. There are several sources of communication stress and these should be explained to the client.

Thinking/Talking—Propositionality

The more the stutterer has to think and put his thoughts into words, the more difficulty he has. Another way to view this is that the more abstract the conversation, the more difficulty the stutterer will have. You can demonstrate this by having the client count from 1 to 10 (no thinking or propositionality), and then have him tell you how to put the chain back on a 10-speed bicycle. The client will have more difficulty speaking as he attempts to describe this than when counting to 10.

Authority Figures

Authority figures intimidate the stutterer, and he is more likely to stutter. The more authority the person has, the more difficulty the stutterer will have in speaking. Teachers, principals, parents, and clinicians are all examples of figures of authority.

The Number of Listeners

As the number of listeners increases, so does the communication stress. Speaking in front of a class is a good example of this. This also includes speaking situations where there are a number of people who can overhear the stutterer, even though he is not talking directly to them, for example, ordering food in the lunch line. The client must speak more loudly in this situation, and other students ahead or behind him in the line can hear him if he stutters.

Time Pressure

When the stutterer is hurried in his speech, he will have more difficulty in speaking. One of the reasons the telephone [42] is a feared speaking situation is that the stutterer feels he must speak quickly so that the person on the phone knows he is there. This same "time pressure" is present when the client attempts to break into a conversation when a group of people are talking. He finds it very difficult to "get a word in" when there is only a slight pause in the conversation and he feels he must "rush" to break in. There are many sources of "time pressure," some real and some imagined, but the stutterer reacts by attempting to hurry his speech attempt. As a result of the hurried speech and the tension of trying to interject his comment, the probability of stuttering is increased.

Emotional Content of the Speech

When the stutterer is attempting to communicate something of an emotional nature, the chances of his stuttering are increased. It is important to explain that the emotional content can be either positive or negative. The stutterer will have trouble in either communicating a negative message such as explaining why he was late to school or a positive message such as telling his parents that he found $20 in the street. Both positive and negative emotions precipitate stuttering.

Combinations

All of these previously described factors can be combined in a single speaking situation, and most situations have several of these factors. If a stutterer is standing in front of his class and responds to a question, the speaking situation includes thinking/talking, authority figure, the number of listeners, and time pressure stress. There may also be stress from emotional content if the stutterer does not know the answer to the question.

EFFECTS OF STRESS ON SPEECH [41, 61]

The client must be trained to evaluate his various speaking situations in terms of the amount of stress he experiences in them. You can establish this by first determining what the easiest speaking situation is for him. This may be speaking at home or speaking with his friends. You should identify this as a 1 speaking situation. Then determine the most difficult speaking situation, such as reciting in class or talking on the telephone. This would be a 5 situation. After the easiest and hardest situations are determined, find a 3 situation, then a 2 and a 4 situation. All talking situations can be assigned to one of these stress levels. If the telephone is a 5 situation, then any other situation where there is the same amount of stress is also a 5. Have the client relate his speaking situations for the day and attempt to assign them a stress level. Clients in this age group should have no difficulty in learning to assign stress levels to their speaking situations. These stress rating levels will be used when the client begins to use the log book later in therapy.

WHY LISTENERS REACT TO STUTTERING [50, 58]

Explain to the client that, in most instances, he indirectly tells the listener how to react to his stuttering. The listener may not be sure how to react so he looks to the stutterer for clues. If the stutterer is embarrassed and shows it by his facial expressions and other behaviors, the listener is also embarrassed. But, if the stutterer does not show any signs of embarrassment or struggle behavior, the listener will be more relaxed and have a less negative reaction.

EFFECTS OF SPECIFIC SPEECH BEHAVIORS ON STUTTERING

Explain, or even demonstrate for the client, the effects that various speech behaviors have on stuttering. As you explain and demonstrate, have the client imitate you to observe the effect on his speech.

Rate of Speech [43]

Stutterers tend to speak at a fast rate in order to (1) say what they want to say before they stutter or (2) say it fast to get it over with. This fast speech rate creates problems because they do not have time to coordinate their speech mechanisms or time to organize what they want to say. If the rate of speech is reduced, they have more time to do these things. The speech should be at a slow, relaxed, normal rate, but not so slow that it calls attention to itself or interferes with communication.

Explain to the client that people have two speech monitoring systems, one system that monitors their own speech internally, and a second system that monitors the speech of other people, speech from outside. It seems as though the speedometer or timing mechanism of the internal monitoring system is not working properly for stutterers. When they talk at a normal rate it will sound very slow to them, even though it sounds normal to everyone else.

Enunciation [44]

The client should understand that on many occasions he will attempt to say a particular sound but his mouth is in the position to say another sound. For example, the stutterer may want to say the sound (b) but has his mouth open saying the (ah) sound. He could not possibly say the (b) since the lips are parted. The stutterer should have his mouth in the correct position to say the sound he wants to say, even if he does stutter on it.

—NOTES—

Speech is monitored through both auditory and oral sensory cues. Stutterers appear to pay too much attention to the auditory cues and not enough attention to the oral cues. To improve their speech, they must attend more to their oral cues. The easiest way to do this is to have them attend carefully to the cues, to enunciate carefully, or "talk with their lips" as one young stutterer put it.

Easy Vocal Onset [44]

Some stutterers attempt to talk while they are holding their breath. They close their vocal folds very tightly and then try to build up enough breath pressure to overcome the tense vocal folds to produce voice. Easy vocal onset consists of starting the air flow and then closing the vocal folds around the moving column of air. It is somewhat akin to saying a very short (h) before the sound. This is particularly important in the production of vowels. Each vowel should be produced with an easy vocal onset. When easy vocal onset is used it prevents the occurrence of breath holding.

Note. Be very cautious about the concept of the (h) sound being similar to easy vocal onset. The client may adopt this strategy, using an (h) for easy vocal onset. The (h) then becomes a secondary mannerism, a language modifier like an (uh) used to get a word started [45]. Like the (uh), the client then begins to stutter on the (h) sound. The respiratory system is now involved, making the block even more complicated.

Flow of Speech [45]

Explain carefully that most stutterers pause, stop speaking, in order to "get ready" to say words they fear. As a result, their speech flow is fragmented and choppy. Most stuttering occurs when the stutterer initiates speech [40]. Therefore, the more pauses and breaks there are in the flow of speech, the more chances there are for stuttering to occur, since the client is initiating speech again after each stop. The client should flow all of his words together in his phrases in order to minimize the chances of stuttering.

GOALS OF THERAPY [95]

The client should be told the goals of therapy and, according to his age, understand that there is no cure for stuttering. He should understand the difference between "fluent speech" and "normal sounding speech." Instruct the client that if the speech is slow enough there will be no stuttering, the speech will be fluent. Demonstrate this to him at one word per second. He will then understand that, although it is fluent, it is not normal. "Normal-sounding speech" has a normal rate and may even have some very short, effortless prolongations. Listeners would consider this normal speech, not stuttering.

The goal of therapy is controlled fluency. It is designed to meet both of the fears that stutterers have, (1) that the stuttering will occur and (2) that the block will last so long that they will appear foolish to their listener. This means that therapy is designed to first achieve a maximum of fluency through the use of a new speaking behavior. Dysfluencies will still occur in the speech, however they will not resemble the original stuttering blocks. Rather, as long as the client is performing the new speech behaviors (rate, enunciation, easy onset, and flow—REEF), the dysfluencies that occur will be slight prolongation, just a momentary "hangup" of a movement. These are called stickies since the speech movement "sticks" momentarily. In the event the duration of the sticky becomes too long, or if a stuttering block should occur, the client is taught the "glide" [45]. This is the voluntary movement of the articulatory system from the "stuck" position into the next sound. The second technique the client is taught is stop/correct [46]. In the event the glide does release the block, the client stops his speech, backs up a bit and starts again, but now using his REEF. Thus, normal sounding speech is achieved through controlling the fluency through specific speech behaviors, and blocks or long stickies are minimized through the use of the glide or stop/correct techniques.

The client should be told that therapy is designed to reduce the "severity" of stuttering to the point where it no longer is a problem in his life. He must understand that he will still have stuttering blocks occasionally and that he needs to know how to deal with them through the glide or stop/start. It is important to discuss the two basic fears that the stutterer has and how they will be dealt with in the therapy program [95].

GETTING THE NEW BEHAVIOR TO OCCUR

GENERAL CONSIDERATIONS

Goals

The goal of this step in therapy is to create controlled fluency in the clinical environment. With controlled fluency the client will still have very short effortless prolongations (stickies) but they will not interfere with his communication or resemble the original stuttering blocks. The speech will be "normal" for all intents and purposes. The client should also be able to control the duration of either stickies or blocks when they occur.

It is at this point that the client should first begin to realize that he can control his stuttering. This is the beginning of change of the cognitive set from being a helpless victim to taking control of his speech.

Speech Objectives

Behaviors to minimize stuttering

Rate of speech (R) [43]. We want to slow the rate of speech in the client. The goal is not slowing the speech to abnormal rates, but rather to a slow, normal speech rate. This is the rate that you might use when explaining something to a child, a rate of approximately 120 words per minute. We do not want the new rate to sound abnormally slow. This rate allows the client time to coordinate his speech mechanisms as well as time to organize his thoughts.

Enunciation (E) [44]. The client needs to pay more attention to the oral sensory cues, the kinesthetic and proprioceptive cues which tell him what position his articulatory system is in. I have found that most clients understand the term "enunciation." However, with some younger clients I have told them to "talk with their lips" and this seems to convey the concept.

Easy vocal onset (E) [44]. Many stutterers use a hard vocal attack when uttering a vowel or vowel-like consonant. Clients may start their speech with the vocal folds held closed, attempting to speak while they are holding their breath. They should start all vocalization from a relaxed position of the vocal folds, somewhat as if they were using a very small (h) sound before each vocalization. However, it is very important that the client not be taught to use the (h) sound, because he may then begin to stutter on the (h) sound, involving the respiratory system in the stuttering block, increasing its complexity.

Note. The use of easy onset is an option for the clinician. Many stutterers do not need to learn this technique, because they are not having difficulty in initiating vocalization. This technique is specifically for those stutterers who attempt to speak while they hold their breath and push to get the voice started.

Flow of speech (F) [45]. By eliminating the stops and pauses present in the stutterer's speech, we can reduce the probability that stuttering will occur. If most stuttering occurs at the initiation of speech, we can reduce the probability of stuttering by reducing the number of times the stutterer initiates each instance of speech.

Flow also includes a steady flow of speech rather than sudden spurts of rapid speech in what would otherwise be normal speech rate. The client needs to give equal speech time for all words. Many stutterers start speaking with a sudden burst of very rapid speech. If, when they start speaking, they give all words equal time, the probability of stuttering is greatly reduced.

Dealing with remaining stuttering

If the client is using the new speech behaviors (REEF), the dysfluent episodes which remain will not be the "hard," struggling blocks which characterized his stuttering before therapy. The remaining dysfluencies will be effortless prolongations, usually lasting less than 1 second. These are referred to as stickies rather than blocks since the articulators seem to just "stick" for a moment. When the sticky terminates, a glide occurs naturally, with the client gliding into the next sound of the word. It is important that the client learn to perform to glide intentionally.

There is no way that you can be assured that the client is going to use his REEF effectively in all of his speaking situations. When his controls are not working effectively, he will have some stuttering blocks, although they will not be as severe as the blocks he had before therapy. In order to terminate the blocks and gain control over his speech, he can use the glide or the stop/correct technique. The client should first try the glide; but if that fails, he should then use the stop/correct technique. In some very difficult speaking situations where the REEF is not working effectively, the stickies may increase in duration to the point where they begin to interfere with the flow of speech. The stutterer should then glide out of the sticky in order to shorten it.

The glide [45]. The glide consists of a reduction of the speed of transition of the articulators from one sound position to the next. The client purposely moves his articulators slowly from the "stuck" position to the next sound in the word. Once the client learns to use the glide he can glide through those words that he fears he might stutter on, initiate his speech by gliding into the first word, or shorten long stickies by gliding out of them.

Stop/correct [46]. Another technique the stutterer may use in dealing with a stuttering block is to stop the speech attempt and start over again, the stop/correct technique. It is extremely important that the stutterer recognize that if he stops and begins again, *he must begin again using his speech controls, his REEF.* The block occurred because he was not using his REEF. Therefore, if he stops, he must begin again using his speech controls and employing the glide on the word he stuttered on. If he starts his speech again, using the same speech behaviors as before, this is a "retrial," a secondary mannerism where the stutterer simply repeats the lead-in phrase in hopes that the stuttering will not occur again.

Group and/or Individual Therapy [81–83]

It is probably more efficient to teach new speech behavior in individual therapy. However, teaching can also be accomplished in a shaping group. In essence, you would be doing therapy in a group by working individually with the client in a group setting. One advantage of teaching the new behavior in a group setting is the strength of the rewards the client receives from a peer group [86].

The Clinical Stimulus Roles [27–29]

The clinician. During this phase of therapy we want to establish two stimulus roles in the clinical environment. By rewarding the new speech behavior we become associated with the rewards and assume the role of S+. This role then assists in therapy by cuing the new speech behavior to occur when we are present. As the new behavior becomes more predictable and occurs more often, we then begin to penalize the occurrences of the old behavior. Through this association, we become an S- , cuing the client not to produce the old behavior since it will result in penalty.

Other clients. If the therapy is being performed in a shaping group, the members of the group will assume the same roles as the clinician as they administer rewards for the new speech behavior (S+) and penalties for the old behavior (S-).

Parents. Prior to the client's coming in for therapy the parents have established stimulus roles through the reward. If they rewarded the stuttering by being solicitous or overly attentive, their S+ role maintained the stuttering. If they penalized the client for stuttering they maintained it through the heightened fear and anxiety they created. In order to start an effective therapy program we must change their stimulus roles to an S0, eliminating the influences that are maintaining the stuttering [40].

THERAPY PROCEDURES

An Overview

The therapy interaction in this phase of therapy is based on the CIM [23–26] and is directed at teaching the client the new behaviors of slower rate of speech, using careful enunciation while speaking, using easy vocal onset in speech, and flowing the words together to eliminate unnecessary pauses: REEF [43]. These behaviors are taught to eliminate as much stuttering as possible. We are teaching the client a new way to speak which includes all four behaviors, the REEF. *These are all taught simultaneously and constitute the client's new speech behavior which results in controlled fluency.* The client is then also taught how to use the glide and stop/correct techniques [45–47] in order to deal with remaining stuttering blocks which, since the client is not cured, will still occur.

The process that will be used in therapy is that of shaping. The new speech behavior will have to be taught over time, shaping the client's behavioral responses closer and closer to the behavioral goal by rewarding more successful performances [31]. The most convenient way to reward the client is to work in a token economy [31]. This is particularly true if therapy is being performed in a shaping group.

If a DAF unit is available, you can use it to teach the new speech behavior. However, the behavior can also be taught using modeling, guidance, and information. In using either technique, you will provide most of the modeling, guidance, and information for the client, even in a group setting [19]. However, as the new speech behavior begins to occur, rewards can be given either by the you or by the members of the group [20, 85]. It is the occurrence of the new behavior that is rewarded, not the resultant fluency [43]. The fluency is only a by-product of the use of the new speech behavior.

The therapy interaction initially consists of modeling, guidance, and information; but as the client becomes more familiar with the new behaviors the interaction changes from a teaching mode to a practice mode and the assistance you provide is faded [20]. To enable the client to practice the new behavior, the interaction should be conversational in nature. The topic of the conversation must be carefully controlled in terms of communication stress [41]. Manipulation of topics to increase communication stress is used in the next phase of therapy to test the stability of the new speech behavior.

Therapy Steps

A. Start therapy by giving the client an appropriate stimulus which will lead to the performance of the new speech behavior you want to teach. You will be changing an existing speech behavior that contributed to stuttering to a new form which is conducive to fluent speech.
B. Carefully evaluate the client's responses and respond accordingly. If a response shows some positive movement toward the behavior change goal, reward the client. If the response demonstrates no change, respond to the client in a relatively neutral way, for example, "Let's try it again." Each transaction is a test to see if the client learned what you were teaching. Penalty is not used early in therapy.
C. Start succeeding transactions based on your evaluation of the client's response. If the response indicated a positive change in behavior, proceed to the next step in teaching the behavior. If the response was not satisfactory, repeat the transaction. Modify your stimulus to give the client more information about the behavior you want to occur.

D. If there is a series of unsuccessful transactions, closely examine the client's attention to therapy (his motivation), the appropriateness of your stimulus, and the appropriateness of your rewards and penalties.

E. As therapy progresses, raise your standards of acceptance for the behavioral response of the client, rewarding only the better productions. When the client is able to produce the new behavior in some form, introduce penalty for occurrences of the old behavior or for poor productions of the new behavior. You are now encouraging production of the new behavior and discouraging production of the old behavior.

F. As the client becomes better able to perform the behavior, slowly reduce the amount of modeling, guidance, and information you are providing. Your stimulus should shift to a more conversational mode, allowing the client to produce the behavior independent of cues from you.

G. Continue to reward all occurrences of the new behavior. Toward the end of this phase of therapy the use of penalty should no longer be necessary since the old behavior is no longer occurring and the performances of the new behavior are more consistent.

H. When the client performs the new behavior 90% of the time in the clinical environment with no cues from you, move to the next phase of therapy.

Teaching the New Behavior

The clinician's stimulus [19]: Without a DAF unit

Modeling. Start by demonstrating the new speech behavior and having the client imitate you. You will probably have to exaggerate the rate and enunciation for the client initially, but as the client learns to imitate the REEF speech, you can make your model more natural. In order to get the flow, you may have to work with the client on phrasing. You might start with three-word phrases and work your way up to longer, more natural phrases where there are no pauses or stops. As the client successfully models your speech, the glide should occur spontaneously. Do not be alarmed if the client speaks very softly when he is first using the new behavior. As he becomes more comfortable with it, the normal loudness will return.

Should the desired behavior occur in a shaping group where another group member has achieved the speech behavior you are teaching, you can use this group member to model the new behavior for the client.

Guidance. There are two forms of guidance you will use with this client. As he attempts to imitate your speech model you will give him gestural guidance in the form of gestures to prompt, for example, slower speech, or more enunciation. You might also give him verbal guidance, using words such as "slower," "enunciate," and "flow."

Information. You can give the client behavioral information during all of his attempts to imitate your speech model. Initially, describe what REEF speech sounds like. Carefully describe the speech in terms of rate, enunciation, easy onset, and flow. As you progress in getting the new behavior to occur, you will continue to give the client information about how to refine it. As the glide occurs, provide more information about how it is performed and how it is used in controlled fluency. You can also provide information on the use of the stop/correct technique.

Stimulus manipulation [29–31]. There are many stimuli in the client's environment which might interfere with his ability to perform the new speech behavior. You can exert some control over these stimuli to assist the client. If you are working with the client in a group, you may find that he is unable to perform the new speech behavior in front of the other group members; there are too many stimuli, too much pressure [41]. You might have to work with this client outside the group in order to get the new behavior to occur. The topic you choose to talk about is also a matter of concern. If the topic is too sensitive he may not be able to produce the new behavior. Choose a neutral or pleasant topic to discuss as he attempts to imitate your speech model.

As the new speech behavior begins to occur and results in controlled fluency, point out to the client that he is creating the controlled fluency by using the new speech behavior. This is a major step in changing his cognitive set [49, 56–65].

The clinician's stimulus [19]: With a DAF unit

Before introducing delayed auditory feedback (DAF), give the client some instructions on how to speak while using the unit. Instruct him to talk slowly and speak very carefully, to enunciate his words. Tell him that you will help him do this by giving him guidance while he is speaking, using hand gestures that mean slow down, enunciate, easy onset, and flow.

Before putting on the earphones, turn on the DAF and let him hear the "echo" so he knows what to expect when he has the earphones on. Depending on the type of DAF unit you have, set the delay time somewhere between 0.200- and 0.250-ms delay time. Be certain that you have turned down the volume of the unit before putting the earphones on the client. You can then have him read or talk about something as you turn up the volume. How loud should it be? Loud enough so that the client's bone conduction hearing is masked. It must be quite loud but not painful. Try it on yourself to gain an idea of where the control should be set. If it is not loud enough, the client will be able to hear himself and you will not get the DAF effect.

At first, the speech may be worse than it is without the DAF. Have the client continue talking as you provide gestural guidance to slow him down, use more enunciation, and so forth. Continue this process until the speech becomes fluent. This may take anywhere from 1 to 10 minutes. Make a tape recording of the client's speech during this time.

If your client can not initiate vocalization as he attempts to speak on the DAF, you will not get the DAF effect. There must be vocalization. If you encounter this situation, teach him the glide so he can get his speech started. Once he is able to start speaking, the DAF effect will occur.

You can teach your new speech behavior goal using the DAF. Not only is the speech rate reduced, the client automatically shifts to enunciation. The easy vocal onset and flow of speech will also occur while the client is speaking on the DAF. If you cannot get the client to flow his speech, have him count slowly and connect all of the numbers together. You should model the counting procedure for the client so he understands he should not stop speaking between numbers.

After the client has achieved the new speech behavior while on the DAF, remove the earphones and have the client use the new speech behavior as he talks to you. You may have to continue using your gestural cues in order to maintain the speech behavior. A word of caution: The DAF effect may last for several hours with the stutterer being very fluent, but this is *not* permanent and the client should know this.

Once you have the new speech behavior occurring, you should ask the client how he is talking differently. Get him to recognize, either from his ongoing speech or the tape recording, that he is talking more slowly, using more enunciation, using easy vocal onsets, and that his speech is flowing together. This new way of speaking should be discussed at length so that the client understands that he is creating the new speech by using his new speaking behavior (REEF) [43]. It is extremely important that the client realize that he is controlling the fluency, it is not just happening. This is another step in changing the client's cognitive set [49, 56–65].

At this time you might also play back the tape recording of the client after he had adjusted to speaking on the DAF. Allow him to hear the recording of his new speech behavior. Point out occurrences of the behaviors in REEF as they occur. This recording is very important to you since it will be used to play back to the client from time to time to remind him of how he changed his speech behavior in order to control his fluency. Do not be concerned if the speech is quite soft when the client first uses new speech behavior. Normal loudness will return as the client becomes more familiar with the new way of speaking.

If your are doing this in a shaping group, inform the other members of the group of what the client is attempting to do. The group members can provide strong rewards to the client as he works on the DAF if they know what the behavior change goal is.

The client's cognition [16]. As the client perceives your stimulus (modeling, guidance, information, or the DAF) he must cogitate or think about it, and then attempt to produce the behavior requested by you. If he can not understand what you expect of him, your stimulus is not appropriate; it may be beyond his ability to comprehend. You must adjust your stimulus to the cognitive level of the client so that he is able to understand what you are presenting to him. His ability to produce the requested speech behavior is directly related to his ability to perceive and comprehend your stimulus.

The client's response [16]. When the client responds he will be attempting to produce the speech behavior that you are teaching. He will monitor his speech as he responds, trying to imitate your model, and adjusting his speech according to his perception of the information you gave him about new speech behavior, or trying to imitate his speech when he was on the DAF.

Note. You can assist the client to perform the requested speech behavior by providing him with gestural guidance, cues, or prompts related to REEF during his response.

The clinician's cognitions [20]. The response of the client is the stimulus you will respond to. As the client responds, you will make four decisions about the response. You will make decisions about correctness, frequency, attention, and the direction of the next transaction.

1. The correctness of the response. This is an indication of whether or not the client is learning the new behavior and if you are going to reward or penalize him. The behavior should improve with successive trials.

2. The frequency of occurrence of the response. If you are using an appropriate reward for the production of the new behavior, it should occur more often. This is your test of the reward you are using.

3. The client's attention to therapy. If the client is motivated he will be attending to therapy. The rewards and penalties you use will have a great influence on the attending behaviors of the client. If your rewards and penalties are not appropriate, the client may lose motivation for therapy and not attend to what you are doing. If this is the case, you will have to change your rewards and/or your penalties.

4. How you will start the next transaction. If the client is learning and the behavior is continuing to improve, you may proceed with your therapy in the next transaction. However, if the speech behavior is incorrect, you will have to repeat the transaction, changing your stimulus. It may be that the client needs a better model, more guidance, or additional information. Your next transaction depends on the results of your testing the current transaction.

The clinician's response [20–23]. There are three possible responses you can give to your client: a reward, a penalty, or no response at all. It is very important that you respond to the client, and the responses you give to your client during this phase of therapy should be primarily rewards. Rewards create approach motivation (and attending behaviors) in the client. The rewards presented during the learning period should be on a continuous schedule.

Penalty should be introduced only after the client is able to produce some form of the new behavior you are teaching. It does not have to be perfect but it should be an approximation of the new behavior goal. Once the client can produce this approximation you can discourage the production of the old behavior through penalty. Penalty also provides the client with avoidance motivation, to not perform the old behavior in order to avoid receiving a penalty.

Rewards [20–22]. Since behaviors that are rewarded occur more often, and you want to encourage the client to use his new speech behavior, reward him each time he uses it. However, be careful in selecting a reward. A contingent event is only rewarding if the behavior being rewarded increases in frequency of occurrence. You must decide, before you start therapy, what you are going to use for a reward. You might ask the client what he thinks would be a reward for him or, in a shaping group, what the group might find rewarding. Discuss this with the clients and make them a part of the decision-making process. A response by you or group members is rewarding only if the client sees it in that light.

Later in this phase of therapy you may find that, as the client becomes more adept at performing the new speech behavior, he may be able to concentrate on a single behavioral element, usually enunciation, and this alone will result in the new speech behavior occurring and the resultant controlled fluency.

Schedules of rewards [21]. You will use a continuous reward schedule in this phase of therapy. In order to achieve rapid learning of the new behavior, this is the best schedule to use.

Penalties [22]. If a client performs the old speech behavior, you should give him some sort of feedback that the behavior is not correct and ask him to repeat it using the new speech behavior. This is a form of penalty. However, you must be certain that he can perform the new speech behavior before you penalize the occurrence of the old behavior. The penalty used does not have to be harsh. For example, you might say to the client, "You did not use your new speech behavior that time. Now, try it again and see if you can use it when you talk this time." The reward is encouraging the new speech behavior to occur and the penalty is discouraging the old speech behavior from occurring.

Changes in Cognitive Set

Clients in this age group usually have well-established negative cognitive sets about their stuttering and themselves. Their cognitive set should be dealt with very directly. In this stage of therapy the client must learn that he is able to change his stuttering for the better. If he has had previous therapy and failed, he may have a negative set toward trying therapy again. The best way to deal with the client's negative set is through success and rewards. However, it is important that you emphasize with the client that *he* is changing the stuttering. Point out carefully that you are only teaching him what to do but that he is the one actually doing it. Dwell on his successes, no matter how small they may be. Praise his attempts to change the stuttering through the new speech behavior. Your reward system is extremely important in changing the client's cognitive set.

To make changes in the client's cognitive set, use these techniques: provide more information about stuttering [56], have the stutterer create a list of assets [60], explain the listener's reaction [58], and do some counseling [59]. Even though you have gone over some of this in the previous phase of therapy, it bears repeating.

Home Program

The home program for this phase of therapy consists of removing those factors in the home that might maintain the stuttering. The most obvious factors are the parents' rewards or penalties for the child's stuttering, which may be working against us as we attempt to create new speech behaviors in therapy. We should also recognize that the influence of the parents and the home program varies according to the age of the client. The information you derived from the initial evaluation and the conference with the parents will help you make a decision about the value of a home program.

Remove rewards for stuttering. If the parents are in some way rewarding the client for stuttering, you must remove the reward if you are going to be able to establish the new speech behavior. You should instruct the parents to ignore, as much as possible, the stuttering in the home and if they do this, you can change their stimulus role for the old behavior from an S+ to an S0 [29]. To accomplish this, you will have to work on the parent's cognitive sets [65, 69].

Remove penalty for stuttering. Some parents may be penalizing the client for stuttering in the home, which creates many negative attitudes in the client and interferes with your attempt to create the new speech behavior. The parents need to be instructed that the penalty is making the stuttering more severe and that they should try to ignore the stuttering in the home. At this point in therapy, you can change their stimulus role from an S- to an S0 for the old behaviors [29], and also begin to change the cognitive sets of these parents [65,69].

Monitoring the home program. You must monitor the home program very carefully by creating a reporting system. The parents must keep you informed about what is happening in the home. This communication could be in the form of conferences, telephone calls, or written reports, depending on the time you have available. The parents are emotionally involved with their child [65, 69] and, not being trained clinicians, they will need a great deal of supervision with the home program.

Working with Teachers

If you can get cooperation from the client's teachers, you will deal with them much as you did with his parents. You want to eliminate, as much as possible, any actions by the teachers that might reward or penalize the client's stuttering. Therefore, you should provide them with some information about stuttering in order to change their attitude toward the client's stuttering and modify their reactions to it. An information sheet for teachers is included in Appendix E. This form can be changed according to your own unique situation and sent to teachers whose actions might be interfering with therapy. It is important to get this information to the teachers early in therapy, because you may wish to call for their assistance in later phases.

STABILIZING THE NEW BEHAVIOR

GENERAL CONSIDERATIONS

Goals

Our goal is to stabilize the new speech behavior and the resultant controlled fluency in the clinical environment. We want the new behavior to occur without cues or prompts from us and with no specific reward from us. The client should be able to maintain his controlled fluency with no direct assistance from us.

In terms of the client's cognitive set, he will now begin to realize that he can control his speech to the point that it is "normal" in the clinical environment.

Speech Objectives

(a) During this phase of therapy we want the client to be able to use his new speech behavior [43] consistently without our assistance, either from prompts or from rewards. There should be approximately a 90% reduction in the number of stuttering blocks that he would have had.

The blocks should be replaced by stickies with no emotional involvement or struggle behavior. The number of stickies and their length will vary according to the emotional stress the client is under in the clinic room.

(b) The client should be able to use the glide or stop/correct [45] to deal with all of the remaining stuttering blocks. He should first attempt to glide out of the block, but if this fails, he should stop, go back a couple of words, and start again using his REEF, and then glide on the word he stuttered (the stop/correct technique).

Group and/or Individual Therapy [81-83]

It would be best to work with the client in this phase of therapy in a shaping group. The client needs to be able to use his new speech behavior in a social situation. The shaping group provides him with an opportunity to verbally interact with other children and to enter discussions of various topics. He also needs to learn that he can speak to peers without stuttering and, thus, influence his cognitive set [80]. The new speech behavior can also be stabilized in individual therapy, but it is more difficult because he is gaining experience in talking with only one person, not a peer, which does not allow for social interaction.

The Clinical Stimulus Roles [27-29]

The clinician. The stimulus roles we established in the first phase of therapy are now to be altered. Our role of S+ fades to that of an S0 as we remove the reward for use of the new behavior. By the end of this phase of therapy we should assume the S0 role, indicating that we will not reward the occurrences of the new behavior. If the new behavior is stable it should not be affected by the removal of the rewards. Since the old behavior is no longer occurring, our S- role has also shifted to an S0 since we are no longer penalizing the old speech behavior.

Other clients. The other members of the shaping group assumed the same roles as the clinician in the first phase of therapy. They will also shift their roles to that of an S0 as they remove their rewards for the new behavior and penalties for the old speech behavior. Their stimulus role parallels that of the clinician.

Parents. It is now time to involve the parents actively in the therapy program. As the new speech behavior becomes more stable in the clinical environment, you want to have the client begin to use it at home. The parents should be instructed to reward the client when he uses his new speech behavior at home. As they reward the client they become an S+ for the new speech behavior. As the new behavior is stabilizing in the home, the parents can begin to penalize the old speech behavior, becoming an S- for stuttering behavior.

THERAPY PROCEDURES

An Overview

The CIM continues to be the basis of clinical interaction [23-26]. We are not involved in teaching the new behavior in this phase of therapy, rather we are providing the client with an environment where he can practice using the new speech behavior while speaking on a variety of topics and, if he is in a group situation, while interacting verbally with a group of peers. As we move into this phase of therapy, the performance of the new behavior is dependent on the rewards the client receives in therapy. However, we now begin to slowly remove the rewards, changing our reward schedule from a continuous schedule to an intermittent schedule [21].

The shaping process [31] is still being used, although we are now shaping the new speech behavior to occur in different conversational modes and while speaking about different topics. We increase emotional content as the new behavior becomes more stable [41]. We cannot move out of this phase of therapy until the client can maintain his new speech behavior regardless of the topic in therapy, and without prompts or rewards from the clinician or other group members. If the rewards are withdrawn too rapidly, the performance of the new behavior may slip. In this event, increase the rewards until the new behavior is back to where it should be and then begin to remove the rewards again, but remove them more gradually.

Therapy Steps

A. Therapy in the early stages of this treatment phase is reward oriented. The new behavior is still dependent on the rewards and there should be no drastic change in the reward schedule as you move into this phase. You briefly continue with a 100% reward schedule, then shift to rewarding approximately 90%, 80%, and so forth until the rewards are eliminated.

B. Monitor the client's new speech behavior carefully to determine the effect of the removal of the rewards. If the speech deteriorates, it means that the new behavior is still dependent on a certain amount of reward. In order to get the new behavior back to the appropriate level, increase your rewards. Once the new behavior is again stabilized, start fading the rewards again.

C. Your transactions with the client are now mainly in a conversational mode. You are prompting speech through questions, requests for information, or other such stimuli. You are providing the client with an opportunity to practice his new speech behavior in a social context, in a conversational mode. Your transactional testing now focuses on the stability of the new speech behavior as the rewards are slowly withdrawn.

D. All transactions are still dependent on the results of the preceding one. If good controlled fluency is maintained as the rewards are removed, continue to remove them. If the speech proficiency drops, reevaluate the reward and reward schedule.

E.   As therapy progresses, continue to decrease the number of rewards the client receives. When the client is able to maintain his new speech behavior 90% of the time, regardless of the topic of conversation, with only an occasional positive comment by your or a group member, you are ready to move to the next phase of therapy.

Stabilizing The New Behavior

The clinician's stimulus [19]. To stabilize the new behavior, your clinical focus is to give the client an opportunity to practice his new speech behavior while speaking about a variety of subjects. Your stimulus will be framed in such a way as to elicit as much speech as possible from the client. Avoid asking questions that can be answered in one or two words. Ask the client to tell you about something or describe something. You might ask him to tell you about a vacation, to describe a movie or television program he has seen, to tell you about his hobby, and so forth. Keep the topics of conversation rather neutral early in this therapy phase. As the new behavior becomes more stable and you are able to remove some rewards, increase the complexity of the topics. You can now have him talk about more emotional issues, such as telling you about how other people used to react to his stuttering. You will be applying communication stress [41] to the client to see how well he can manage his speech behavior under these conditions.

The client's cognition [16]. Because you are now requiring the client to converse on various topics, he is going to be attending more to what he is saying than how he is saying it. He will still be thinking about the rewards for performing the new behavior but not to the degree he was in the previous phase of therapy. Further, as therapy progresses and there are fewer rewards, there will be less attending to the performance of the new behavior.

The client's response [16]. The client's response is now conversational. He is thinking primarily of what he is talking about . If he is using his new behavior he will be demonstrating controlled fluency. There will be stickies in the speech, and stuttering blocks may also appear. The client should deal appropriately with the blocks during his speech response. You will gradually eliminate the cues and prompts you provided during the client's responses in the last phase of therapy.

The clinician's cognitions [20]. Your stimulus is the client's response, his conversational speech. The decisions you will make are:

1. The correctness of the response. If the client is performing the new speech behavior, he will be demonstrating controlled fluency. You will have to keep some sort of count or record of your rewards of the new behavior in order to gradually remove the rewards .

2. The frequency of occurrence of the response. The new speech behavior should be consistently performed, not mixed in with periods of occurrence of the old behavior.

3. The client's attention to therapy. Since you are withdrawing your rewards from the client, his motivation for therapy may decrease. However, if the controlled fluency is a rewarding experience for him, this should compensate for the rewards you are no longer giving.

If the client is not attending to therapy, you can focus your therapy on this factor by penalizing nonattending behaviors and/or rewarding attending behaviors. This temporary refocusing of your therapy will not disrupt your stabilization of the new speech behavior.

4. How you will start the next transaction. While you are in this phase of therapy you will continue to provide the client with an opportunity to use the new behavior in a conversational mode. However, as the behavior becomes more stable and independent of the rewards, you should increase the communication stress that the client is experiencing so that he can learn to cope with more stressful talking situations.

The clinician's response [20–23]. Though you will start this phase of therapy with a continuous reward schedule, you will soon shift to an intermittent schedule. You will then gradually withdraw all rewards for performance of the new behavior. In the event that you must work on the client's attention to therapy, you may continue to reward attentive behaviors.

Penalty should be only a small part of your interaction in this phase of therapy. The old behavior should not be occurring except in rare instances when a more emotional topic is introduced. If some stuttering does reoccur, it should not be severe or last for any length of time. If it persists, penalty should be applied to the client if he failed to use the glide or stop/correct techniques since use of these would result in controlled fluency. If the client is having great difficulty in achieving controlled fluency, you may have moved into this phase of therapy too soon.

Rewards [20–22]. The reward that you are using with the client may lose its rewarding effect. The client may lose interest in it or become satiated with it. If the speech behavior begins to falter as you are withdrawing the reward and, even when you increase the reward the behavior does not improve, your reward has probably lost its effectiveness. In this case you will also see a lack of motivation and an increase in nonattending behaviors. You will have to determine another form of reward and then test it to see if it is truly rewarding [20].

If the client is receiving therapy in a group, carefully identify for the other group members what the new speech behavior is that the client is performing for rewards. Also, instruct the group that the client is not going to be rewarded every time he performs the new behavior [22]. You might even arrange it so that the group members would only reward the client at a signal from you. This would give you better control over the reward schedule.

Schedules of rewards [21]. You now shift to an intermittent reward schedule. You use this schedule of rewards because it resists extinction, the fading of the new behavior after the rewards have been removed.

Penalty [22]. Penalty is now directed more at the client's failure to use his controls when stuttering occurs. You do not penalize the occurrence of stuttering. Stuttering blocks will continue to occur since you cannot cure the client. However, he does have techniques to control the stuttering episodes when they occur, and he is penalized when he fails to use them.

Changes in Cognitive Set

This is a very important phase of therapy for changes in the client's cognitive set. It is during this time that the client learns that he can use the new speech behavior and speak with controlled fluency in social interactions. He also learns that he can produce the new speech behavior without having to be rewarded by the clinician or the other members of the group. He is gaining confidence that he can change his stuttering to normal sounding speech. Perhaps the most important thing he is learning here is that *he* can control his speech in social interactions and in discussing any given topic.

During this time the stutterer's self-confidence should increase dramatically. As the fear of stuttering reduces, so will word fears and situational fears. These gains in positive cognitive set are somewhat limited, since he can only use the new speech behavior successfully in the clinical environment.

You will also work directly on changing the cognitive set by giving the client additional information about stuttering [56] and listener reactions [58]. You may also have the client make a list of assets [60] and do some counseling [59]. This would supplement your general comments and rewards in therapy, which are also influencing the cognitive set.

Home Program

You are now ready to start an active therapy program in the home. Having shifted the parents to an S0 in the last phase of therapy, you will now shift the parents to an S+ for the new behaviors. Later you will also introduce the S- role to the parents as they begin to penalize the old speech behavior when it appears in the home.

Providing rewards for new behaviors. The new speech behavior is going to begin to appear in the home. To increase its probability of occurrence, have the parents reward the new behavior, shifting their stimulus role from an S0 to an S+ for the new behavior [29]. This will be a gradual shift of roles for the parents, to be accomplished by the time you complete this phase of therapy. Again, you will have to work on the parents' cognitive sets to have them perform this task for you [65, 69].

Provide penalties for stuttering. You will also introduce the parents to the S- role, penalizing the client for the old behavior when it occurs in the home [28]. This role will not be introduced until the new behavior is occurring rather consistently in the home. You must carefully counsel the parents on what penalty to use, how to use it, and the purpose of the penalty [22]. The parents' cognitive set toward the client's stuttering must be considered and changed if necessary [65, 69].

Monitoring the home program. It is extremely important that you know what is happening in the home program, and the parents should keep you informed. You need to know how often the new speech behavior is occurring, under what conditions, how the parents are responding, how the client is responding, and so forth. In essence, the parents are performing therapy with the client in the home. They are in the first phase of therapy, getting the new behavior to occur, but now getting it to occur in the home. The client knows how to perform the new behavior, but he has no experience with performing it in this environment. His habitual method of speaking in this environment is stuttering, and it will be difficult to overcome this habit pattern and introduce the new behavior.

Telephone calls, conferences, or written reports are the most common avenues of communication. Perhaps the most convenient would be to have the clinician and the parents send notes with the child. If this is supplemented with a few telephone calls, you should be able to establish adequate communication to monitor the program.

Working With Teachers

If the new speech behavior occurs in the home, it probably also will begin to appear in the classroom. And, as with the parents, you would like to have the occurrences rewarded so that they might appear again. You should attempt to enlist the aid of the client's teachers if at all possible. You will not be asking them to perform time-consuming tasks. Rather you would ask the teachers to verbally reward the client when he uses his new behavior. You should caution them not to do this in front of the class but to tell the client after class. This is all you would request of the teacher. You would not introduce penalty for the old behavior in this aspect of your therapy program.

If you have not already sent the teachers information on stuttering, then do it now. The information sheet in Appendix E can be modified to fit your purposes. With this information, the teachers should be able to provide you with some valuable assistance.

GENERALIZING THE NEW BEHAVIOR

GENERAL CONSIDERATIONS

Goals

The goal in this phase of therapy is to get the new speech behavior and the controlled fluency to occur in all talking environments outside the clinic room. We want the client to carry over the new speech behavior into his everyday life and be able to maintain his normal-sounding speech in all speaking situations. We will also begin to focus on training the client to be his own clinician.

It is at this point of therapy that the client comes to realize that he can control his speech in all talking situations. This is a major change in his cognitive set, the point where he begins to realize and believe that he does not have to go through life being afraid of stuttering.

Speech Objectives

(a) Our speech objectives are essentially the same as in the previous phase of therapy except we now want the client to use the new behavior in all talking situations. As the new behavior becomes more stable in other environments, we would expect approximately a 90% reduction in the number of stuttering blocks that he would have had before therapy. We also expect the majority of blocks to be replaced by stickies. The degree of success in carrying over the new speech behavior will be directly related to the stress of the situation where the client is using his new behavior [43].

(b) As before, we expect the client to use the glide or stop/correct techniques to deal with stuttering blocks when and if they occur [45]. These controls, used in conjunction with the new speech behavior [43], should result in normal-sounding speech in all talking situations the client encounters.

(c) We want to increase the number of S+ in the client's environment [27, 30]. We can do this by shifting S- situations to S+ through gradual introduction of the situations [30].

—NOTES—

Group and/or Individual Therapy [81–83]

This phase of therapy lends itself to either group or individual therapy. The client is now speaking with controlled fluency in the clinical environment. The main focus of therapy now is to have the client report on his use of the new speech behavior in outside speaking situations. He can report this to the clinician in individual therapy or to the members of a shaping group. Individual therapy gives you more opportunity to analyze his reports, but the group would be able to provide better rewards and motivation to work on the new speech behavior outside the clinic room. This is an important factor since rewards are now being given for work outside rather than on the new speech behavior in the clinical setting. The rewards, particularly from peers, will have a positive influence on the client's cognitive set [85]. Penalty can also be used in either group or individual therapy. The penalty is not directed toward the new speech behavior (unless needed) but is used to make certain that the client is working outside therapy. If he is now doing his assignments, penalty from a peer group will have a greater impact than from you.

Group therapy also offers you an advantage if the client is faced with a talking situation that is so frightening that he cannot use his new speech behavior when he is in it [28, 30]. If this occurs, you can role play the situation in the group in order to reduce the fear of the situation to the point where the client can deal with it more effectively [81].

The Clinical Stimulus Roles [27–29]

We are now at a crucial point in therapy regarding conditioned stimuli. The client is using his new speech behavior in the clinical environment partially because there are so many S+ cues. He is "reminded" or prompted to use the new behavior whenever he sees the clinician or any members of the group, since they have rewarded him for doing it in the past. We must now attempt to create as many S+ outside the clinic room as possible so that the new behavior is prompted to occur when the client is in different environments. We also need to shift former S− situations to S+, which will prompt the new behavior rather than the old one.

The clinician. We will continue our S0 role for the client's new speech behavior. However, we will reward him for his use of the new speech behavior in outside talking situations, becoming an S+ for work outside the clinic room. We will also assume an S− role if we have to penalize him for not attempting to use his new speech behavior when out of the clinical environment.

Other clients. If the client is working in a shaping group, the other members have assumed the role of an S0 for the new behavior. If the client reports on his outside activities to the other members, they will assume the same roles as the clinician; an S+ for the outside work and an S- if the client is not doing all of his assignments.

Parents. By this time the parents' role as S+ for the new speech behavior and S- for the old speech behavior has been well established. They are now cuing the new speech behavior to occur. As the old behavior occurs less often, their role as an S- fades. During this phase of therapy the parents maintain their S+ role for the new behavior. Their role is extremely important as we introduce the new behavior to environments such as restaurants, stores, friends' homes, and so forth.

Other people and objects. The more S+ you can create, the easier it will be for the client to use the new speech behavior outside. You already have the other members of the group who function as an S+ whenever the client sees them in school. If you can get a teacher to reward him when he uses the new speech behavior (privately, of course), over a short period of time that teacher will also become an S+. If you can get the client to agree, you might have him bring in a close friend who could give the client rewards. This is a good S+ but be careful, since, if their friendship terminates, this could be misused. We can also have objects as an S+. The log book, which is discussed next, will become a very important S+.

The Log Book [60–64]

The log book provides the client with a means of recording the successful practice of his new speech behavior. It is your only major source of information regarding the carry-over of the new behavior to outside talking situations. Clients who stutter have a tendency to remember and dwell on only their speech failures. The log book forces them to recognize their successes. It also serves to remind the client to practice the new behavior so that he can become more proficient. The client may also begin to include speech "games" in the log book at this point, including in his report how long each game lasted. The analysis of the data in the log book is crucial. You must point out the successes he has had both in terms of the reduction of stress in situations and in improved speech performance. It is your main clinical tool in this phase of therapy.

The Telephone [42]

The telephone should be given special attention at this time. It is a main source of social interaction, and, if the client is afraid to use it, he has a significant social handicap. It is a unique talking situation, because there is no direct contact between the people involved in the conversation. The stutterer feels he must respond quickly so the other person on the telephone knows that he is there. The time pressure involved in talking on the telephone makes it one of the most feared talking situations among stutterers. For more specific information on the stutterer's fears associated with the telephone, see Leith and Timmons (1983). A special program for working on the telephone is presented in Appendix F.

THERAPY PROCEDURES

An Overview

The new speech behavior is now occurring, but not where needed, in talking situations outside therapy. You must transfer it to other talking environments. You will now shift the focus of your therapy to the antecedent events, that is, the various S+ and S- in the client's life. You must manipulate these stimuli so that new S+ encourage the new behavior to occur, and shift the S- talking situations to either an S0 or an S+. Therapy will focus on stimulus control [27–31].

You are now asking the client to give reports, written and oral, on how well he is able to use his new speech behavior outside the clinic room. Your stimulus to the client is usually in the form of asking for information. If the client has had a problem with a particular talking situation, you provide him with information as you explain why he had difficulty [41]. The interaction is highly cognitive as the client discusses his talking experiences in other environments. He is given many rewards for his outside work and his success in using his new behavior.

You are still shaping the new speech behavior, but you are now concerned about its occurrence in situations with differing amounts of communication stress. You explain to the client that he will be able to use the new behavior in easier talking situations better than in more difficult ones [41, 61]. The most important aspect of therapy now is to develop some way the client can record his attempts to use the new speech behavior in other talking situations. To record these attempts you will use the log book [60–64]. You should make specific assignments as to the number of times you want him to practice his new behavior each day and instruct the client to start his practice in easier situations in order to increase the probability of success.

Therapy Steps

A. As you move into this phase of therapy you are no longer rewarding the speech behavior in therapy. You now have to introduce the client to the idea of practicing his new speech behavior outside of therapy. You explain that, as with baseball, you have to practice to learn how to use new behavior. You also have to explain the difference between a *practice* and a *game*. Your therapy will consist of evaluating the client's speech efforts outside therapy.

B. After you have introduced the client to the log book, you will have to check it during each therapy session to see if he understands what you want him to do. You may have to explain the log book carefully several times before he totally understands it. Even if the records in the log book are incorrect at first, you should reward the client for his efforts. It is these rewards that will make the log book an S+ for the client.

C. When the client is recording his speech practices correctly, carefully review them with him [63]. Find something positive in each one so you can reward his effort. Point out better speech grades and any reduction in the fear of talking situation. Reward his willingness to practice as well as the success he has when he uses the new speech behavior. It is very important that he understands that his speech behavior will be better in easier talking situations than in more difficult ones. Have him practice in easier situations early in this phase of therapy so that he will have more success.

D. The clinical transactions are now focusing on the client's cognitive set. You are emphasizing his successes in using his new speech behavior. If there is a situation where he thinks he failed (the new speech behavior did not occur) you can still reward him for his willingness to practice. There is no such thing as a failure with a reported situation, only varying degrees of success.

E. As you proceed in this phase of therapy, have the client practice his new behavior in more difficult situations [41, 62]. He may have limited his practices to talking to his friends and family. Have him work up to practicing in more difficult situations such as answering a question in class. Move slowly so that the practices are successful.

Generalizing The New Behavior

The clinician's stimulus [19]. Your stimulus now is most often in the form of questions about the client's practicing of his new behavior outside therapy. Request that he give you a report from his log book. With some of the more successful practice situations you may ask him to give you more detail so you can provide additional rewards. Discuss the situations with him in some detail. If he has a question about a situation or his speech, give him information about it. Ask him if the new behavior is occurring spontaneously in his everyday speech. When this begins to occur, this can also be rewarded.

An important new aspect is now introduced into your stimulus. This is in the form of an informational question [20]. When the client has had a successful practice, you may want to begin the next transaction by asking him why his speech was so good in the particular situation. If he answers by saying he does not know, you must pursue this until he understands that the controlled fluency was a result of his using his new speech behavior. He must realize that he is the person who is making the speech normal sounding. It may take three or four transactions before this is clear to the client, but it is vital that he recognizes that he is controlling his speech. This is one of the most important aspects of the client's cognitive set that you must change, that is, his feeling that he is helpless about his stuttering.

The client's cognition [16]. An important part of your therapy is the client's cognitions about his speech. You are providing evidence through the log book that he can successfully perform the new behavior outside therapy and produce normal-sounding speech. His cognitive set has been changed somewhat in previous phases of therapy, but it is at this point that he learns he can control his speech in all talking situations. It is here that the client learns to trust his ability to control his speech. This is where his confidence is built up, his new self-concept is formed, and where his fears decrease. You are now working more with the stutterer than the stuttering.

The client's response [16]. The client now responds to your questions about his outside speech practice. As he tells you about his experiences and his reactions to his speech, you will hear a reflection of his cognitive set. If he centers only on the negative aspects of his practices, this is a reflection of his negative set. You should counter this with the positive aspects of the situations. If he reports that the new behavior is beginning to occur in his speech outside his practices and games, this is important information for you since this indicates that the new behavior is stabilizing outside.

The clinician's cognitions [20]. You will be attending more to what the client is telling you than to how well he is using his new speech behavior during the report. If the client is using his old speech behavior in his reporting, you might remind him to use his new speech behavior. Should this occur repeatedly, carefully consider whether the client should be in this phase of therapy. During the client's reports, evaluate correctness, attention, and direction of the transactions.

1. The correctness of the response. You are most interested in the client's interpretation of how well he did in his practices and if he did all of his assignments. Although you are not rewarding his speech behavior in therapy, you are involved in rewarding his practicing outside or penalizing him if he fails to do his assignments.

2. The frequency of occurrence of the response. The log book and the reports tell you how often the behavior occurs outside the clinical environment, and particularly if it is occurring spontaneously in the client's general speech, not just during practices. The rewards for the client are very important here. Rewards come from you as you review the log book and from the success the client is having with the new speech behavior. If the new behavior is not increasing in frequency of occurrence, review the type and amount of reward the client is receiving.

3. The client's attention to therapy. The client's attention is still an extremely important part of your therapy. Since you are providing the client with rewards you should be able to maintain his motivation and attention. Some problems with motivation and attention may arise, since he will be facing feared talking situations. If an S- situation is so frightening that the client cannot deal with it, you might role play this in therapy to weaken the fear. Problems with motivation in this phase of therapy are usually related to the client's fear of talking situations being stronger than the motivation to practice the new behavior.

4. How you will start the next transaction. Starting the new transaction will depend on how much information you want from the client from each situation and how the client interpreted the situation. If the client is unaware of how successful he was in a situation, you might want to expand on this by giving him information about his success. You might even want to discuss a particular situation in more detail. When you feel that you have all the information you need and the client has all of the information you want to give him, move ahead in the next transaction.

The clinician's response [20–23]. Your response should consist of rewards for practicing the speech behavior outside therapy. The rewards should increase the probability that the speech practice will continue. You may also occasionally reward the client for his controlled fluency when reporting to you, but this should not be the focus of your rewards.

If you use penalty, it should be used for not completing the practices you have assigned or for using the old behavior without using the glide and/or the stop/correct techniques. No penalty should be associated with the actual practices, only the failure to complete the practices or to record them properly.

Rewards [20–22]. Your rewards in this phase of therapy should supplement the rewards the client is receiving from his new controlled fluency. The main problem you face in generalizing the new speech behaviors is that your rewards are not contingent to the behaviors. You should work with the client's log book so that he will associate the reward with practices and the successes he has had.

If the client is reporting on his practices in a shaping group, point out the client's successes to the group and have them reward the client. Even though you may have to carefully structure the group, it does not weaken the reward [86]. The reward from the peer group is very strong and will help motivate the client as he takes his new behavior out into new environments.

Schedules of rewards [21]. You are now going to have to shift back to a very heavy reward schedule. The client will need as much reward as possible for practicing his speech outside the therapy room.

Penalty [22]. Penalty is now directed to failure to complete outside assignments or for using the old behavior and not controlling it during reports to you. Avoidance motivation will be a valuable adjunct to the approach motivation the client already has. If the client is reporting to a shaping group, the peer penalty will be very strong and will create avoidance motivation. This should result in all assignments being completed.

Changes in Cognitive Set

It is at this stage of therapy that the client finally realizes that he can control his speech and have controlled fluency in all speaking situations. Major changes in cognitive set occur here. In analyzing the log book, you should stress the fact that the controlled fluency is occurring only because the client is performing his new speech behavior. He must come to realize that he is the one who is controlling the speech and that he can do this in any talking situation.

The client's self-confidence should increase. However, you now have to deal with the client's speech goal, making it realistic and achievable. It is not uncommon for the client to have a goal of perfect speech. You must establish with the client a goal of normal-sounding speech, pointing out that normal speech is not perfect. You might have the client listen carefully to nonstutterers and make note of the pauses, breaks, repetitions, and other dysfluencies that occur in their speech.

Another thing you must deal with is that the stability of the client's controlled fluency will vary according to the stress he experiences in various talking situations [41]. His speech will be better in easier speaking situations. He must accept the fact that he has not been "cured," but that he can produce speech that is normal sounding in all of his talking situations. He will have the most difficulty in 4 and 5 situations. However, as he gains confidence, he will have fewer of these situations and, even when he is in one, he will be able to produce better speech. Dealing with the client's speech goal and his acceptance of less than perfect speech is important as you change his cognitive set and expectations from therapy.

With many clients you will have to supplement your use of the log book to change cognitive set with other techniques such as discussing listener reaction [58] and making a list of personal assets [60]. Counseling [59] can also be of value here since the client is now interacting with listeners outside therapy and encountering new and more challenging talking situations.

Home Program

The home program is extremely important here. The parents are now S+ for the new speech behavior and an S- for the old behavior. The client should now be performing the new speech behavior rather consistently in the home. The parents can also help in generalizing the new behavior to other environments by taking the client with them on shopping trips, to friends' homes, and other social activities. Their presence as an S+ in these talking situations should prompt the new speech behavior to occur so it can be rewarded. They are also of valuable assistance in reviewing the log book with the client. They provide an important support system to the client as he begins to use his new speech behavior outside therapy and the home environment.

Providing rewards for new behaviors. The parents should be providing rewards for the new speech behavior when it occurs in the home or in other environments. Their role as an S+ is especially important outside the home where they prompt the new behavior to occur there. They should also reward the client for his work on the log book and reward his efforts to practice. The log book becomes a very strong S+, since both you and the parents reward the reports from it. Because the client carries the log book with him at all times, it serves to prompt the new behavior to occur and to remind the client to use his new speech behavior.

Provide penalties for stuttering. Once it is established that the client can produce the new speech behavior in the home, penalty should be administered when the old speech behavior occurs. Again, the parents should be counseled on the penalty to use and the purpose of penalty [22]. As the speech behavior becomes more stable in the home there will be less need for penalty for the old speech behavior.

There should also be penalty associated with failure to practice the new speech behavior and record it in the log book, just as you are doing in therapy. This penalty is not associated with the speech behavior but with the failure to practice it.

Monitoring the home program. Monitoring is an extremely crucial point in therapy, and good communication between you and the parents is vital. You must know how well the client is doing in using his new behavior in the home and in other environments. You also need to know how the parents are responding to the log book as they review it with him. In the early stages of this phase of therapy you will be primarily concerned with the performance of the new speech behavior in the home, but, as therapy progresses, your concern will shift to the client's speech performance in other environments. The information you receive about the client's performance in the home program will prove to be a valuable supplement to the information you have available in the log book.

Working With Teachers

You can now expect the new speech behavior to occur with greater regularity in the classroom. One of your tasks in this phase of therapy is to increase the number of S+ to prompt the new behavior to occur in different speaking situations. The client's teacher is a valuable S+ at this time. She can assume this role by simply rewarding the client when he uses his new behavior. If she is consistent in her rewards, telling him after class how well he did, she will quickly assume this role. Do not introduce penalty in this situation.

To accomplish this, you will need to have a conference with the teacher and explain exactly what behavior the client should perform in order to be rewarded. If this is the first time you have approached the teacher, you should provide her with the information about stuttering for the teacher in Appendix E. However, if the teacher was involved in the previous step of therapy, you need only to ask her to continue but explain the new goals of this phase of therapy.

MAINTAINING THE NEW BEHAVIOR

GENERAL CONSIDERATIONS

Goals

In this final part of therapy, our goals are to eliminate all clinical contact with the client and to complete training the client to be his own clinician. He must be able to continue to deal with his stuttering without our support or input.

In terms of the change in the client's cognitive set, it is here that he learns that he not only has control over his speech, but he also has the responsibility for it. He must learn to trust himself to act as his own clinician.

Objectives

(a) The client should be able to analyze his own log book and recognize the importance of specific accomplishments in the various practices. He should be able to judge how many practice situations he will need each week in order to maintain the new speech behavior.

(b) The client should be able to recognize when and if his performance of the new speech behavior is slipping and to decide what he should do to improve it. He needs to understand how to go about strengthening his new behavior should it begin to fade, and the role of the log book in accomplishing this.

(c) He should know how to deal with new and stressful speaking situations. He will meet new situations as he matures and he must feel confident that he can deal with them.

Group and/or Individual Therapy [81–83]

The client is phased out of all regular clinical contacts in this part of therapy. His activities during the time he is in therapy are focused on his reports of his use of the new speech behavior in outside environments. Most of this information will come from his log book. His reports can be presented in either group or individual therapy. Group therapy would have the advantage of peer rewards for a good report and penalty for failure to work on his speech [85]. Individual therapy would have the advantage of more individual guidance as the client assumes more and more of the responsibility of acting as his own clinician.

The Clinical Stimulus Roles [27–29]

The clinician. We continue to be an S0 for the new speech behavior in the clinic room. If the speech begins to falter, we can provide the client with some rewards and/or penalties, but this should not be a continuing activity. If rewards and penalties must continue over a period of time, the client should be taken back a step in therapy; we moved too fast. We are now assuming an S+ role for his being his own clinician, rewarding his insights into problems he might have had and his method of dealing with them. We might also assume an S- role if the client is failing to perform as his own clinician.

Other clients. If the client is a member of a shaping group, the members play the same roles as the clinician, an S0 for the speech behavior and an S+ for the role of being his own clinician. When the client is rewarded for a report from his log book, he is also being indirectly rewarded for using the new speech behavior in practices.

Parents. The parents also have to shift their roles and the behaviors they have been rewarding. They are an S0 for the client's speech behavior but they now must develop the S+ role for the behavior as a clinician. They might also assume the S- role if the client fails to act as his own clinician. If this occurs consistently, they should inform you so that you can reevaluate where he should be in the therapy program.

The Log Book [60–64]

The client has used the log book to practice his new speech behavior so he could speak in any situation with controlled fluency. He now needs to practice the new speech behavior in order to maintain it. You can draw an analogy in sports with a professional baseball player. He first has to practice batting to learn to be a good batter. Once he becomes an outstanding batter, he has to practice in order to maintain his batting skill. This same principle applies to the field of music. When a person practices to become very good at a special skill, he/she must practice to maintain the skill. Just playing in concerts or in baseball games is not enough to maintain the skill.

The client also has to practice to maintain the new speech skill he has learned. Just talking games are not enough to maintain the skill. The client must keep his log book going, doing one practice a day to maintain his skill. There is always self-doubt in the cognitive set of the stuttering client, and the record in the log book will do wonders to counteract the self-doubt and maintain the self-confidence.

THERAPY PROCEDURES

An Overview

The time has come to gradually withdraw direct therapy contacts from the client. There should also be less and less input from us [30]. We will allow the client to take a greater responsibility for both his speech and the meetings, either individual or group, where he reports on his outside speech achievements. He is not *given* answers to problems he might face, he is allowed to plan a strategy, which we discuss with him. Our goal is to train him as a clinician and we do this not by forcing decisions or strategies, but by allowing him to think through the problem and discuss it with us. We do not relate to him as a client, but more as a clinician discussing a client. Some of the contacts with the client should probably be on an individual basis but they do not need to be long conferences. Ten minutes should be adequate.

We start this phase of therapy by reducing the therapy contact with the client by 50%, seeing him once instead of twice a week. We then move to seeing him once every 2 weeks, and so forth. If he falters in his role as clinician, we can always increase the clinical contact to stabilize this new behavioral role.

Maintaining The New Behavior

The clinician's stimulus [19]. When you see the client, ask him questions about his experiences outside, and provide him with information when he asks for it. Lead him to answers to problems rather than providing them for him. This is an important part of the training.

The client's cognition [16]. The client is now thinking about how well he is performing his speech behavior in outside speaking situations. He will also be involved in attempting to resolve any problems he might have encountered in using the new behavior outside therapy. His cognitions should now be those of a clinician who is working with a client.

The client's response [16]. The client's responses reflect his evaluation of his speech outside therapy. He should be reporting and asking questions. In many instances the CIM appears to be reversed, with the client providing the stimulus of a question or statement and you responding. This will occur more often as he assumes the role of being his own clinician.

The clinician's cognitions [20]. You will be evaluating either the client's stimulus if he starts a transaction or his response if you have initiated the transaction. You continue to make decisions although they are now slightly different.

1. The correctness of the response. You now judge the correctness of the response in terms of the client's role as a clinician. This determines whether you reward him for his role as his clinician or penalize him for failing to perform. The influence of your reward or penalty is directly related to how often you see him in therapy. If the correctness of the behavior is a consistent problem, you have to take the client back to the previous phase of therapy.

2. The frequency of correctness of the response. You have to judge not only how well the client is functioning as his own clinician, but also how often he is doing it. You have very little direct control over this, and if it presents a continuing problem you will have to back up one step in therapy.

3. The client's attention to therapy. You no longer have any significant control over the client's attentiveness to his speech behavior and his role as clinician. If he is not attending you will see the effects of it in the first two decisions you make and should act accordingly.

4. How you will start the next transaction. When you initiate the next transaction you will either be asking for more information, providing an opinion, or leading the client to more appropriate solutions to problems he is facing [10–12]. These transactions are rather loosely structured since they are more conversational than transactions in any other phase of therapy.

The clinician's response [20–23]. Your rewards will be focused on the behaviors associated with being a clinician. You will reward the client's insights into problems, his solutions to those problems, his awareness of his speech behavior, and so forth.

Penalty should be used only if the client is failing to assume the role of being his own clinician or not performing the role frequently enough.

Rewards [20–23]. Your rewards now are going to be limited in their effectiveness due to the periods of time between clinical contacts. The stronger you can make the reward, the longer its effects will last [21]. Relating to the client as a clinician (rather than a client) should provide him with some reward. It is a challenge to develop adequate rewards in this phase of therapy. You can only hope that the controlled fluency the client is experiencing is providing sufficient rewards to maintain his motivation.

The group continues to be a source of strong rewards by peers. The group members must be aware of what behavior they are to reward. You may have to manipulate the group in order for rewards to be applied to the appropriate behavior [86], since the new behavior (acting as a clinician) is more subtle and not directly related to speech.

Schedules of rewards [21]. You should provide as many rewards as possible to the client. It will be impossible to maintain a continuous reward schedule because of the type of relationship you now have with the client, but you should stay as close to the continuous reward schedule as possible.

Changes in Cognitive Set

The client has learned that he can control his speech in all speaking situations, but he must now learn to assume total responsibility for his speech. He has been dependent on other people, especially you, up to this point, but he now must learn to deal with his speech by himself. The client must learn to trust himself as a clinician. This is a new concept for the client, and he will need support from you as he takes on this role. His comfort with the role and his trust in himself as a clinician will come with successful speech in outside speaking situations. He is already doing this, but has not yet realized that he can do this by himself, without guidance from you.

As the client begins to realize that he can act as his own clinician, the added self-confidence will be reflected in changes in attitudes and beliefs about his stuttering. He will begin to develop a strong positive cognitive set and this should result in behavior changes such as the client's becoming more assertive, more verbal, and more socially oriented.

Home Program

The home program will continue to focus on generalizing the new behaviors to other speaking environments. The progress made in the home program should increase as we complete training the client to be his own clinician. This will result in the client's being less dependent on the parents for support. As the new speech behavior is generalized, the parents will be able to gradually withdraw their rewards, shifting their role back to an S0 [29].

You will not be able to include the parents in training the client to be his own clinician. There are too many factors involved, which are often too subtle for the parents to observe and reward. Further, the insights and strategies for which you are rewarding the client call for a professional understanding of the stuttering problem and the role of the clinician, which the parents do not have. The client, being a stutterer and having observed you function as a clinician over a period of time, has insights that are limited to persons who stutter or who are professionally trained clinicians.

Working With Teachers

The classroom teachers cannot assist you in training the client to be a clinician. They can continue to reward the speech, but this continuing reward should not be necessary. The training of a clinician calls for special insights and knowledge which the classroom teacher does not have.

References and Recommended Readings

Ainsworth, S. (1975). *Stuttering: What it is and what to do about it.* Lincoln, NE: Cliffs Notes, Inc.

Belgum, D. R. (1974). *What can I do about that part of me I don't like?* Minneapolis: Augsburg.

Bloodstein, O. (1975). *A handbook on stuttering.* Chicago: National Easter Seal Society for Crippled Children and Adults.

DeVreugd, P. (1982). *The physiological loci of stuttering blocks in children.* Master's thesis. Detroit: Wayne State University.

Gregory, H. (1973). *Stuttering: Differential evaluation and therapy.* New York: Bobbs–Merrill.

Hill, W. F. (1971). *Learning: A survey of psychological interpretations* (3rd ed.). Scranton, PA: Chandler.

Kübler-Ross, E. (1969). *On death and dying.* New York: MacMillan.

Lefrancois, G. R. (1972). *Psychological theories of human learning: Kongor's report.* Monterey, CA: Brooks/Cole.

Leith, W. R. (1971). Clinical training in stuttering therapy: A survey. *Asha, 13,* 6–8.

Leith, W. R. (1979). The shaping group: Habituating new behaviors in the stutterer. In N. J. Lass (Ed.), *Speech and language: Advances in basic research and practice* (Vol. 2). New York: Academic Press.

Leith, W. R. (1982). The shaping group: A group treatment procedure for the speech/language clinician. *Communicative Disorders, 8,* 103–115.

Leith, W. R. (1984). *Handbook of clinical methods in communication disorders.* San Diego: College-Hill Press.

Leith, W. R. (In press). The stutterer with atypical cultural influences. In K. St. Louis (Ed.), *The atypical stutterer.* New York: Academic Press.

Leith, W. R., & Chmiel, C. C. (1980). Delayed auditory feedback and stuttering: Theoretical and clinical implications. In N. J. Lass (Ed.), *Speech and language: Advances in basic research and practice* (Vol. 3). New York: Academic Press.

Leith, W. R., & Mims, H. A. (1975). Cultural influences in the development and treatment of stuttering: A preliminary report on the black stutterer. *Journal of Speech and Hearing Disorders, 40,* 459–466.

Leith, W. R., & Timmons, J. (1983). The stutterer's reaction to the telephone as a speaking situation. *Journal of Fluency Disorders, 8,* 233–243.

Leith, W. R., & Uhlemann, M. R. (1972). The shaping group approach to stuttering: A pilot study. *Journal of Comparative Group Studies, 3,* 175–199.

Levis, D. J. (1970). *Learning approaches to therapeutic behavior change.* Chicago: Aldine.

Martin, G., & Pear, J. (1983). *Behavior modification: What it is and how to do it.* Englewood Cliffs, NJ: Prentice-Hall.

Meichenbaum, D. M. (1977). *Cognitive behavior modification: An integrative approach.* New York: Plenum.

Norman, D. S. (1969). *Memory and attention.* New York: Wiley.

Perkins, W. H. (1973). Replacement of stuttering with normal speech: I. Rationale. *Journal of Speech and Hearing Disorders, 38,* 283–294.

Perkins, W. H. (1978). *Human perspectives in speech and language disorders.* St. Louis: Mosby.

Riley, G. D. (1972). A stuttering severity instrument for children and adults. *Journal of Speech and Hearing Disorders, 37,* 314–322.

Speech Foundation of America. *Counseling stutterers.* Publication #18, Memphis, TN.

Speech Foundation of America. *If your child stutters: A guide for parents.* Publication #11, Memphis, TN.

Speech Foundation of America. *Stuttering: Its prevention.* Publication #3, Memphis, TN.

Van Riper, C. (1982). *The nature of stuttering* (2nd ed.). Englewood Cliffs, NJ: Prentice-Hall.

Westberg, G. E. (1962). *Good grief.* Philadelphia: Fortress Press.

Appendix A

LOG BOOK: INSTRUCTIONS

1. Any time you speak to someone you can use this as a practice situation for your log book. Asking a friend a question, ordering food in the lunch room, calling a store on the phone; all of these can be practice situations. To make these into practice situations you must plan *exactly* what you are going to say before you go into the situation. By doing this, you do not have to think of *what* you are going to say since you will already have it memorized. In that you must memorize what you are going to say, your "practice" will not last more than 10 or 15 seconds. During this time you are to concentrate on using one part of your new speech behavior, such as a slower rate of speech or enunciating as you speak. You should practice all of the parts of your new speech behavior as you use your log book.

2. The first thing you enter into your log book is something that will remind you of what the situation was so that you can remember the situation when you talk to me about it. You might enter such things as "Called Fred," or "Answered question in class."—just enough information so that you can remember the situation.

3. The second thing you write down is how much "stress" you think you are going to have in the talking situation. Rate the "stress" you expect on the 5-point scale we talked about where a 1 situation is a very easy talking situation and a 5 situation is a very hard situation.

4. Write the first two things in your log book before you go into the talking situation. This is very important since we need to know how much stress you *think* you are going to have in each situation. After you have written this in your log book, plan exactly what you are going to say and what you are going to practice. You can then go into the situation.

5. After you have finished saying what you have memorized, write down how much stress you feel after having done the practice. This is the *actual* stress that you had in the situation. For example, you might have written down a 4 stress before asking a question in class. But, since

you planned what you were going to say and practiced a new behavior, your speech was very good. Because your speech was good, your stress level after the situation was only a 3. The stress level after the situation may be higher, remain the same, or go down. Write down your stress level after you leave the situation.

6. The fourth thing you should write in the log book is a "grade" for your speech in the situation. You will use the following grading system:

A—speech was very good with no blocks. There were some small stickies in the speech but they were hardly noticeable. The listener considered you a normal speaker.

B—speech was very good with no blocks. There were some longer stickies in the speech. The person listening may have noticed them but they did not disrupt the speech. The listener considered you a normal speaker.

C—speech was still good with no blocks. The stickies were longer and disrupted the flow of speech. The person listening to you noticed the stickies but, since there was no struggle or pushing the words out, considered you a dysfluent normal speaker, not a stutterer.

D—speech was interrupted by some blocks. The blocks were shorter and easier than in the old stuttering and most of the blocks were modified by using the glide or stop/correct techniques. The listener considered you a stutterer but not as severe as you used to be.

E—speech was the same as before therapy. You had no control over your speech and could not practice what you had planned to.

7. The last thing you will enter into your log book will be what behavior or behaviors you were working on in the situation. Your note book should look like this:

1. Asked question in class
2. 4
3. 3
4. B-
5. Rate

1. Called Tom about notes from class.
2. 2
3. 2
4. A-
5. Enunciation

After using the log book for a while, try your new speech behavior in a conversation where you do not have an opportunity to plan out everything you are going to say. Get into a conversation with a friend and see if you can use your new speech behavior during the entire conversation. This is a test of how well you have learned the new speaking behavior. You should enter these game situations into your log book the same way as a practice, but be sure to indicate that the situation was a speech game and write down how long the game lasted.

Appendix B

INFORMATION FOR THE PARENTS OF A STUTTERING CHILD

Dear _____:

Your child is now receiving speech therapy for (his/her) stuttering. I would like to share with you some information about stuttering so that you will better understand how to deal with the stuttering when it occurs in the home.

Most stuttering starts early in a child's life, usually between 3 and 5 years of age. We do not know exactly what causes a child to begin to stutter. All children have interruptions in their speech as they learn to talk. Most children do not pay any attention to the interruptions but others become frustrated by the interruptions and try to change them. They do "tricks" like trying to push words out, whispering, stomping their feet, or hitting their leg to make the interruptions shorter. At first, a trick works and the interruptions are shorter or may not even occur. But in a short period of time, the trick does not work any more, and the interruptions get longer and occur more often. So, the child tries another trick. It also works for a period of time and then the interruptions come back. The child eventually becomes frightened because he finds that, no matter what he does, the interruptions keep coming back and they are occurring more often and lasting longer. When the child becomes frightened about his speech and the interruptions, he is stuttering rather than having the normal interruptions found in children's speech. The interruptions are now stuttering blocks. His speech is blocked. He cannot say a word even though he knows exactly what he wants to say. The more frightened he becomes, the more the blocks occur, and the more the blocks occur, the more frightened the child becomes. He then uses more and more tricks to get out of the stuttering block but they all fail after a short period of time. However, the child does not stop doing a trick after it no longer works. He just adds another trick. So, over time, the stuttering becomes very complicated.

Children who stutter do not do this on purpose. They do not want the stuttering to occur but they do not know what to do to prevent it from happening. They are embarrassed by it. To avoid being embarrassed by the stuttering, the children do not talk as often or use long sentences.

They use as little speech as possible so they will not stutter. They become afraid of certain sounds and words. They then avoid using the sounds or words so they will not stutter. They also learn to be afraid of certain speaking situations, such as talking in class, and they avoid getting into the speaking situations. It is very common for children who stutter not to answer questions in class because they might stutter and embarrass themselves. They would rather pretend they do not know an answer than to take a chance on stuttering in front of their classmates.

How should you react when your child is stuttering to you? *First,* you should look directly at your child while he is stuttering and make no comments, just wait for him to get out what he is trying to say. If you look away or try to say the word for him, you only make him more embarrassed and the stuttering will get worse. *Second,* you should not hurry your child while he is speaking. If he tries to speak faster there will be even more stuttering. *Third,* you should be as relaxed as possible while with your child. The more tense he is, the more he will stutter. He will also stutter more when he is excited, since this is another form of tension. *Fourth,* you should not express your frustration with your child's speech, either verbally or through your facial expression, since this will only make him more nervous and he will stutter more.

Appendix C

STUTTERING THERAPY WITH CHILDREN WITH OTHER HANDICAPS

It is not uncommon for a client who stutters to also be learning disabled, mentally retarded, hearing impaired, or have some other problem. This does not prevent you from providing clinical services for the stuttering. The therapy presented in this book is still applicable, but you will have to modify certain aspects of the CIM to account for the other handicapping condition. Depending on the particular problem, you may have to modify your stimulus or your response, or monitor the client's attending behaviors carefully. The changes or modifications you might have to make in the CIM are as follows.

The clinician's stimulus. You may have to adjust your stimulus to the perceptual or cognitive level of the client. With an auditory perceptual problem you will have to be cautious when using auditory stimuli. You must make certain that the client is perceiving your stimulus, since if he is not perceiving it, he can not comprehend it. Your stimulus will also have to be adjusted for those clients who have a cognitive problem. You must make sure the client comprehends what you are saying. With both the perceptually and cognitively handicapped client you should continually verify his comprehension of your stimulus. You can do this by asking the client for information, having him repeat back to you what you have just told him. If he did not comprehend your stimulus you will have to repeat the informational transaction, modifying your stimulus. You may have to expand your stimulus to other sensory channels; providing the client with a more detailed stimulus including modeling, guidance, and information and utilizing the auditory, visual, and bodily sense channels.

The clinician's cognitions. The second adjustment you may have to make in the CIM concerns your evaluation of the client during the clinical transactions. In addition to evaluating the speech response, you are going to have to carefully monitor the client's attending behavior. If the client is highly distractable, you must make some adjustments for this. You can deal with this to some degree with your rewards but this may not solve the problem. You may also have to modify your clinical environment, removing as many distracting stimuli as possible and covering up those which cannot be removed. The client must be attending to your therapy if any learning is to take place.

The clinician's response. You may have to modify your rewards and penalties according to the handicapping condition of the client. If the client is emotionally impaired, you should be cautious about the types of rewards you use, and consider carefully the use of penalties. You do not want to aggravate any emotional problems the client is having by applying inappropriate rewards or penalties. With the cognitively impaired client, secondary rewards such as verbal praise or tokens may have no meaning and, thus, not function as a reward. In this event you will have to use a primary reward such as a food item.

The multiple handicapped client presents some unique clinical problems. As you attempt to resolve these problems, turn to the CIM and it will assist you in analyzing the problem and planning an appropriate clinical approach to the client.

Appendix D

MINI-GUIDE FOR PUBLIC LAW 94-142

The following has been excerpted from *A Mini-manual for Teachers in Special Education Programs* by Dr. Mae Taylor, Specialist in Communication Disorders, Utah State Office of Education, a small and succinct reference for state and federal regulations for public school special educators and speech clinicians. This is not meant to be a replacement or substitute for the more detailed federal document nor for local or state interpretation; it is meant only as a handy reference for the clinician and is an example of one state's document to assist personnel in programs for the handicapped in the schools.

Permission for Testing/Evaluation

1. Permission for testing forms must include the following: (1) areas in which tests are to be administered; (2) names and purpose of the tests in each area; (3) date; (4) signature of the person sending the form to the parents; (5) the reason(s) for testing. All of the above items must be completed prior to sending the form to the parents for their signature.

2. Permission by a parent must be given by a signed and dated signature. If there are boxes, which are to be checked indicating permission or refusal, included on the form, the appropriate box must be clearly checked.

3. Permission for testing shall never postdate the actual testing date.

4. Permission for testing needs to be reobtained only if it is determined that areas will be tested for which existing permission is not now granted.

Diagnosis and Assessment

1. Diagnostic protocols, or summary reports, must be included in a student's folder in order to support the student's classification of handicapping condition.

2. More than one measure must be used to determine classification of handicapping condition. (In the case of an articulation disorder the two measures might be (1) a standardized test of articulation and (2) observation of the student's articulation in conversational speech.)

3. Protocols and reports must be signed in full and dated as to day, month, and year.

4. Testing instruments must be selected so as to measure the student's natural ability and not reflect environmental, sensory (visual or auditory), physical, or ethnic background.

5. Classification must be made by a multidisciplinary team or group of persons.

Individualized Education Program (IEP)

1. Completion of blanks: All sections and spaces contained on the district's/agency's IEP form must be completed (filled in), including (1) the student's classifying information, (2) the student's present levels of achievement, (3) strengths, (4) weaknesses, (5) annual goals, (6) short-term objectives that are measurable.

2. Signatures: The team's complete signatures must be individually dated in full (day, month, year).

3. Classification: Classification must be written out, as opposed to initialed or coded, on the IEP, and fully explained to the parents.

4. Focus on the learning problem: Annual goals and short-term objectives must be focused on the student's problem.

5. Review: IEP's must be reviewed and updated as often as required, but *at least annually.*

Participants in Meetings

1. All IEP meetings conducted for all categories of handicapping conditions must utilize the minimum number of participants: (1) local district or agency representative; (2) the student's teacher; (3) the parent or guardian.

Permission for Placement

1. The IEP spells out or dictates the placement of the student.

2. The IEP must be fully completed *before* placement occurs (services begin).

3. All required information on the Permission to Place form must be completed, including (1) description of placement options considered, (2) reason(s) for proposed placement including the anticipated length of service, (3) name, date, and title of the person completing the form, (4) parental permission must be clearly indicated and signed in full including the date of the signature, (5) other alternatives considered and rejected are no longer mandatory, but remain a good practice.

4. A new Permission for Placement form does not need to be reobtained unless the student's placement option is changed.

5. The permission for placement form must be signed by the parent *before* the student can be serviced.

Termination

1. When it is determined that a student can be released from special education services, the action must be accomplished through the IEP process. The same kind of meeting held to classify the student and write the IEP must be held to declassify.

2. When students move from school to school, or between levels (elementary to junior high to senior high), they are still classified as handicapped unless a declassification meeting is held. If they are not declassified, they must be served. A move between levels is not justification for terminating special education services to the student.

3. When the parents or students refuse the services offered, the agency is strongly advised to provide a form for parents to sign indicating that services have been offered but refused.

Other Required Documentation

Location of documentations listed may vary, depending upon state or district practices.

1. Primary language of the home: The primary language needs to be documented in the student's folder and is frequently placed on the IEP form.

2. Justification for Placement: A justification for the placement option selected is most often found on the IEP form. Options considered must be listed on the Permission for Placement form.

3. Due Process Information Dissemination: Documentation of dissemination of due process information (rights of parents) must be presented.

4. Record of Access: A Record of Access form must be available for use before a student's file is accessed.

5. Access and Authorization: A file access authorization list shall be maintained for public inspection and shall include a full listing of the names and positions of those staff members who may have access to personally identifiable information. The list shall be updated as necessary and shall include the following six categories: (1) name of staff member who has permission to access the records; (2) position of staff member who may access records; (3) name of the district; (4) name of the school; (5) school year in which effective; (6) identification of records manager.

6. Services Mandatory: Any student classified as handicapped for educational purposes must be served—there can be no waiting list.

Appendix E

INFORMATION FOR THE TEACHER OF A STUTTERING CHILD

Dear _____:

A child in your class, _____, is receiving speech therapy for (his/her) stuttering. Stuttering is a complex problem and I would like to share with you some information about stuttering so that you can better deal with the problem in your classroom and, perhaps, even assist me as I attempt to eliminate the stuttering problem.

Most stuttering begins early in a child's life, usually between 3 and 5 years of age. We do not know exactly why a child begins to stutter. All children have interruptions and dysfluencies in their speech as they learn to talk. Most children do not pay any attention to the disruptions but others become frustrated by them and try to eliminate them. They do "tricks" like trying to push words out, whispering, stomping their feet, or hitting their leg to make the disruptions shorter or eliminate them. At first, a trick works and the interruptions are shorter or may not even occur. But over a period of time, the trick no longer works, and the disruptions become longer and occur more often. So, the child tries another trick. This also works for a period of time and then the disruptions return. The child eventually becomes frightened because he finds that, no matter what he does, the disruptions keep coming back, occurring more often and lasting longer. When the child becomes frightened about his speech and emotionally involved in the disruptions, he is stuttering rather than having the normal dysfluencies found in children's speech. The disruptions are now stuttering blocks. His speech is blocked. He can not say a word even though he knows exactly what he wants to say. As he becomes more frightened, more blocks occur; and the more blocks that occur, the more frightened the child becomes. He then tries trick after trick to get out of the stuttering block but each trick fails after a short period of time. However, the child does not stop performing the trick after it no longer works. He just adds another trick. So, over time, the stuttering becomes very complicated with the child repeating a sound over and over, blinking his eyes, nodding his head, stomping his foot, and so forth.

Children who stutter do not do this on purpose. They do not want the stuttering to occur, but they do not know what to do to prevent it from happening. They are embarrassed by it. To avoid being embarrassed by the stuttering, the child does not speak often or use long sentences.

They use as little speech as possible so they will not stutter. They become afraid of certain sounds and words. They then avoid using the sounds or words so they will not stutter. They also learn to be afraid of certain speaking situations, such as speaking in class. *It is very common for a child who stutters not to answer questions in class, even though he knows the answer.* He would rather pretend he does not know an answer than to take a chance of stuttering in front of his classmates. He may also become somewhat of a disruptive influence in the class because he is trying to gain some recognition from his peers. The stuttering child has very low self-esteem, a poor self-concept. He compensates for this by either withdrawing or becoming aggressive and assertive. Underlying all of this is the tremendous fear the child has of appearing "foolish" in front of others, especially his peers.

How should you react when the child is stuttering while talking to you? *First,* look directly at the child while he is stuttering and make no comments, just wait for the child to get out what he is trying to say. If you look away or try to say the word for the child, it only makes the child more embarrassed and the stuttering worse. *Second,* if the child is speaking in class, do not hurry him while he is speaking. If the child tries to speak faster there will be even more stuttering. *Third,* you should be aware of how the other children in the class are reacting to the child. If they are teasing him or laughing when he tries to talk in class, you should deal with this directly. When the child is out of the room explain to the class that he cannot help talking this way and when they laugh and tease him it only makes it worse. *Fourth,* even though it may be frustrating for you when the child is speaking in class, do not show your frustration either verbally or by your facial expression since this will only make him more nervous and he will stutter more.

I would be more than happy to meet with you and discuss this matter. If you would like to meet with me, please contact me and we will arrange a mutually convenient time.

Appendix F

DEALING WITH THE TELEPHONE

When the stutterer gets old enough to use the telephone he will probably begin to develop a fear of it, since he will experience penalty as he stutters while talking on the telephone. If your client has fear associated with using the telephone, you should work on this as part of your therapy. The following is a method of helping your client overcome his fear of the telephone. You should not use this technique until you are into the generalization phase of therapy. Your client must be able to perform the new speech behavior to achieve controlled fluency before addressing the problem with the telephone. You should also recognize that this is usually one of the most fear-provoking speaking situations that the stutterer has, and it will be a difficult task for the stutterer to deal with.

We are going to use the technique of gradual introduction of the stimuli as we deal with the telephone. By this point in therapy, your client should have gained considerable self-confidence in terms of his ability to produce good speech, and this should have resulted in a much more relaxed approach to speaking. However, if we present the telephone stimulus at full strength, have the stutterer sit down and make difficult calls, he may become so fearful, anxious, and tense that he will not be able to use his new speech behavior. We must introduce the telephone gradually. But first, we must teach the stutterer how to relax and how to report his level of relaxation to us.

The technique I use to train the client to relax and to recognize his tension is with an imaginary outside elevator. I have the client close his eyes and furnish an empty elevator as a room where he can relax. We decide on the floor covering, the wall covering, a relaxing chair to sit in, what type of music he would like to listen to, and what he would like to see outside a window in the outer wall of the elevator. I also have the client put a column of buttons on it next to the chair. While the client still has his eyes closed, I ask him to imagine that he is sitting in the chair, looking around the room. I have him "look" at the strip with the buttons and explain to him that there are 15 buttons on it, each of which is a floor number and which lights up when the elevator is at that floor. The top five buttons are red, the next five are yellow, and the bottom five are green. All of this detail is necessary since we must have the client visually imagine and "see" the elevator, to look out the elevator window and listen to the music. He must be attending to these things, not thinking about his problems, if he is going to be able to relax.

When we are through "decorating" the elevator I have the client open his eyes and tell me about the most frightening speaking situation he has ever experienced. When he has identified it, I tell him that this was the 15th floor of the tension elevator. We next decide what his most relaxing experience is, such as listening to his favorite record, watching his favorite television program on a Friday evening, or some other such relaxing experience. This is then identified as the 1st floor of the elevator. I explain that the top floors are red (danger), since he cannot speak well with this much tension. The yellow (caution) floors are a little better, but he must monitor his speech carefully to control it. The green (neutral) floors are comfortable enough that he can control his speech with little effort.

Our next task is to establish where his elevator is at that moment. We know it is not at the 1st floor or at the 15th floor, so we take time for him to decide where his tension elevator is; for example, the 8th floor. When this is determined, I have the client close his eyes and look around his elevator. He is then directed to push the button for the 7th floor. I tell him to signal me by wiggling his finger when his tension is slightly decreased and his elevator is at the 7th floor. I then give him directions on getting his elevator down by telling him to look out his elevator window, listen to the music, and concentrate on the feeling of the elevator descending. I continue giving these cues until he signals that he is on the 7th floor. The process is then repeated several times until we are down to the 3rd or 4th floor. With training the client will be able to reduce his tension by using his elevator without assistance. He will also be able to tell you what tension floor he is on.

Once this is established, I have the client get his elevator to about the 7th floor and then start the presentation of the telephone. If the client's elevator goes up, we stop until he can get the elevator back to where it should be. Once it is back we resume the presentation of the telephone. The following represents a home program for older clients. However, the hierarchies are the same as you would use if you worked directly with the client on the telephone. You may have to simplify the program and the instructions with young clients who fear the telephone. I have used this program with clients as young as 8 years of age.

CALLING ON THE PHONE

Step I

Start this program by unplugging a telephone and taking it to a room where you have some privacy. If you cannot unplug the telephone, tape down the button on the telephone so that when you pick up the receiver you do not hear a dial tone. Just remember to remove the tape when you are through practicing. Now, put the telephone on a table next to a comfortable chair. Sit in the chair and do the following:

1. Get your elevator down to about the 7th floor.

2. Look at the telephone but do not touch it. Just look at it. If your elevator goes up more than two floors, stop looking at the telephone and get back to the 7th floor.

3. When you are back to a 7, look at the telephone again. If you go up more than two floors, stop again and get back to 7.

4. When you are able to look at the telephone and not go over 2 floors, go to the next step and put your hand on the telephone. Again, if the elevator goes up, stop, remove your hand, and get back to 7. When you can touch the telephone and not have your elevator go up more than 2 floors, move to the next step, picking up the receiver but not putting it to your ear.

5. Go through each of the following steps as you maintain your elevator at about the 7th floor.

6. The steps you should go through are:

   a.   look at the telephone,

   b.   touch the telephone,

   c.   pick up the receiver,

   d.   put the receiver to your ear,

   e.   pretend you hear the dial tone,

   f.   dial the first three numbers of a telephone number,

   g.   dial the last four numbers,

   h.   pretend to hear the telephone ring,

   i.   pretend a person answers,

   j.   say "hello," and complete your first sentence.

7. Once you can go through these steps and not go up to the red floors, start making pretend calls to friends (easier talking situations) and then work up to more difficult ones such as calling stores, directory assistance, movies, and so forth. Make a list of five kinds of calls you make and arrange them from the easiest to the hardest. Work your way through your list slowly. Give yourself time to get used to talking on the telephone.

Step II

Now repeat all of the steps using the telephone when it is plugged in or with the tape removed. Do not rush yourself. If you feel your elevator go up, stop and get back to 7 just as you did in Step I. Your telephone calls are real ones now so move very slowly from making easier calls to the more difficult calls.

ANSWERING THE PHONE

The first thing you should do is get someone to telephone you so you can make a tape recording of the telephone ringing. Record about eight rings of the telephone.

Step I

We are going to use almost the same procedure we used with calling on the telephone. Put the telephone, either unplugged or taped, and the tape recorder, on a table next to the comfortable chair. Get your elevator to about a 7 and then turn on the tape recorder and listen to the telephone ring. When you get tense, turn off the recorder and rewind it. Get to a 7 and start it again. When you can listen to it ring about four times and not have your elevator go up more than 2 floors, look at the telephone on the fifth ring. Again, if you get tense, stop and start again.

Using the same procedure, go through the following steps:
    a.   listen to the telephone ring,
    b.   look at the telephone ringing,
    c.   pick up the receiver and turn off the tape recorder,
    d.   put the receiver to your ear,
    e.   wait for about 1 second,
    f.   say "hello."

When you are able to go through these steps without your elevator going up to the red floors, arrange to have a friend call you so you can practice actually answering the telephone. You may have the friend call you several times for your practice. Do not rush to answer the telephone. Take your time and go through the steps you practiced. Since you never know when the telephone is going to ring, you must go through the steps each time you answer the telephone.

Indices
General Index

A

Antecedent event:
  definition, 14
  fading, 30
  (*See also* Clinician's stimulus; Guidance; Information; Modeling; Stimulus manipulation)
Approach motivation (*See* Motivation, approach)
Assets, inventory of, 60
Attending behavior, 17, 24, 75, 91
  (*See also* Behavior, attending)
Attending to oral cues (*See* Enunciation)
Avoidance conditioning, 13, 28
Avoidance motivation (*See* Motivation, avoidance)

B

Behavior:
  attending, 17, 24, 75, 91
    (*See also* Clinical Interaction Model)
  characteristics of, 14, 30, 33–35
  deficit, 34
  definition, 13
  excess, 34
  extinction of, 29
  secondary mannerisms, 36–37
  speech (new), 24
  stickies, 61
  stuttering:
    block, 35–36
    prolongation, 35
    repetition, 35
Behavior change goals:
  eliminate stuttering:
    easy vocal onset, 44
    enunciation, 44

  flow of speech, 45
  rate of speech, 43
  terminate blocks:
    glide, 45
    stop/correct, 46
  (*See also* Controlled fluency; Easy vocal onset; Enunciation; Flow of speech; Glide; Rate of speech; REEF; Stop/correct)
Belgum, D. R., 58
Block, stuttering:
  definition, 35–36
  occurrence:
    linguistic, 40
    phonetic, 40, 57
    physiological, 39
    social, 41–42
  schwa vowel and, 40, 46, 57
  (*See also* Behavior, stuttering)

C

Chimiel, C. C., 44
CIM (*See* Clinical Interaction Model)
Client:
  motivation (*See* Motivation, client)
  response, 16, 24
  seeking therapy, 71–72, 100
  sent for therapy, 72–75
Clinical Interaction Model (CIM), 23–26, 75
  applications, 26
  attending behaviors and, 75
  clinical overview, 26
  counseling and, 59
  model, 25
  shaping group and, 83, 90–91
  speech/attending behaviors, 24
Clinical process, 97–101

—NOTES—

—NOTES—

Treatment Index

—NOTES—